A Neurophysiological Model of Emotional and Intentional Behavior

A Neurophysiological Model of Emotional and Intentional Behavior

By

JOHN L. WEIL, M.D.

Judge Baker Guidance Center
Clinical Instructor in Psychiatry
Harvard Medical School
Boston, Massachusetts

Illustrated by

Gayanne DeVry

and

Elaine Adele Gampp

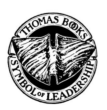

CHARLES C THOMAS • PUBLISHER
Springfield · Illinois · U.S.A.

Published and Distributed Throughout the World by
CHARLES C THOMAS • PUBLISHER
Bannerstone House
301–327 East Lawrence Avenue, Springfield, Illinois, U.S.A.

© 1974, by CHARLES C THOMAS • PUBLISHER

ISBN 0–398–02497–9

Library of Congress Catalog Card Number: 72–88458

Printed in the United States of America

BB-14

Dedicated to

DR. JOHN M. MURRAY

Introduction

The construction of this neurophysiological model of emotional and intentional behavior reflects the goals set forth by D. O. Hebb (1949:xii; 1958:451–66) with respect to establishing avenues of communication between the fields of neurophysiology, experimental psychology, and clinical psychiatry. Hebb has drawn attention to the need for establishing psychological theory upon the basis of current neurophysiological knowledge. He cautions the proponents of behavioral therapy that the central nervous system consists of more than simple circuits directly mediating conditional stimulus-response associations. Likewise he cautions the proponents of psychoanalytical therapy that concepts pertaining to "wishing," "estimating," "judging," and "approving" need to be carefully investigated and defined if they are not to become animistic entities used glibly to explain behavior.

Freud (1954:347–445), recognizing this need to build psychological theory upon a neurophysiological foundation, wrote his *Project for a Scientific Psychology* in 1895. Because of the insufficiency of pertinent neurological information available he was not able to complete his project. However, with the phenomenal advances in the neurosciences over the past twenty years, the construction of a neurophysiological model of emotional and intentional behavior at last may become possible. Success will depend upon the establishment of lines of communication between the neurological and psychological disciplines and the willingness of both groups to profit from reciprocal assistance.

Certain obstacles, however, may hamper communication. The clinically oriented psychologist and psychiatrist may consider reports from the fields of neuroanatomy, neurophysiology, and experimental psychology far removed from an understanding of their patients' emotional problems. Conversely, the neuroscientist has not favored the psychotherapist's subjective concepts and deductive reasoning. However, if the experimental and clinical disciplines are to benefit from an exchange of their experience, and if a theory of human behavior is to be based upon both neurological and psychological findings, it will be necessary for each discipline to work with unusual flexibility to understand one another's language. The psychotherapist must become familiar with important experimental information from the field of neurology, while the neuroscientist must support a quest for operational definitions of subjective psychological terms.

Although the use of deductive reasoning from a number of basic hypotheses has been employed for the construction of the present model's frame, every effort has been made to build the model upon the basis of experimental data. Definitions as far as possible have been formulated operationally. For example, pleasure will be defined as the diffuse perceptual reaction which generally accompanies the activation of central nervous system (CNS) reward mechanisms reinforcing the maintenance of behavior, and displeasure or unpleasure* as the diffuse perceptual reaction which generally accompanies the activation of CNS punishment mechanisms disrupting the maintenance of behavior.

For the psychotherapist who has not been exposed to intensive training in the neurological sciences, a concerted effort has been made to simplify the presentation of complex neurological data. Color diagrams, flow charts, outlines, and tables have been added for the purpose of clarification. It is hoped these aids also will be of value to medical and graduate students who are searching for an outline which will contribute to the understanding of the anatomical relations and functions of the limbic system. Those who are interested in background material will find the inclusion of frequent references to standard texts and reviews of the experimental literature.

Chapters I through IX will focus upon a neurophysiological basis of emotion as a function of upper limbic-hypothalamic-reticular discharge via (1) ascending non-specific activation, (2) descending non-specific activation, (3) extrapyramidal, (4) visceral, and (5) pituitary reactions. The remaining five chapters will deal with a neurophysiological conceptualization of intentional behavior as a function of emotional and cognitive processes. New formulations are presented in Chapters III, VII through IX, and XI through XIV. Other chapters will present experimental detail to establish a scientific basis for these formulations. Since the model is constructed step by step, and one hypothesis is dependent upon another, the reader may best gain an understanding of its meaning by reading the chapters in sequence.

It is hoped the model will stimulate new thought and research both among active experimental investigators and clinicians.

---

* The terms "pleasure" and "unpleasure" parallel "pleasurable" and "unpleasurable"; "displeasure" involves a more limited connotation pertaining to being disturbed and angry.

Acknowledgments

It is a pleasure for me to express my appreciation to all those who have helped in the preparation of this book.

First I would like to thank Mrs. Natalie Stellar for the sensitivity, patience, and wisdom with which she has worked with me to revise and edit the manuscript. The clarity of presentation has without question been enhanced as the result of her skill.

I also wish to thank Dr. Richard Berke whose thoughtful suggestions during the final phase of the manuscript's preparation proved to be most helpful.

During the earlier phases of the work, Doctors Robert Heath, Wallace Tomlinson, John M. Murray, Donald Lindsley, and Dr. Paul Yakovlev generously took time from their rigorous schedules to evaluate portions of the manuscript. To each of these specialists I owe a deep debt of gratitude. Dr. Heath, Dr. Tomlinson, and Dr. Murray offered valuable comments as well as encouragement. Dr. Lindsley raised penetrating questions which led to extensive rewriting of the manuscript. Dr. Yakovlev graciously offered suggestions with respect to the neuroanatomical aspects of the work.

For their interest and help, I want to thank Dr. George E. Gardner, Mrs. Virginia Cirace, Dr. Leston Havens, Miss Arline Husband, Dr. Hugh Leichtman, Dr. Clifford Morgan, Dr. Frank Netter, Dr. Martin Norman, Mrs. Rebecca Norman, Dr. Catherine Roff, Mr. Robert Shilkrit, Mrs. Freyda Siegel, Dr. Samuel Silverman, Mrs. Gertrude Wiseman and Dr. Geraldine Weil.

The "model" was typed by Mrs. Agnes Howard. I have greatly appreciated her most competent and artistic work, and I would like to thank her for her steadfast help and interest over a period of many years.

Miss Gayanne DeVry is responsible for the fine illustrations of the central nervous system. Mrs. Elaine Adele Gampp executed, from the author's original designs, all the diagrammatical illustrations, flow charts, and technical formulae. I am grateful to both of these artists for their excellent work, and additionally appreciate Mrs. Gampp's help and support in taking care of a maze of final details.

To conclude, I should like to thank the staff of Charles C Thomas, Publisher, for their fine cooperation in arranging this publication.

J.L.W.

Contents

xi

List of Tables

A Neurophysiological Model of
Emotional and Intentional
Behavior

Chapter I

Upper Limbic-Hypothalamic-Reticular
Contributions to
Pleasure and Unpleasure

The topic of pleasure and unpleasure reaction has been the subject of dramatic recent neurophysiological investigation and discovery and presents itself as the logical starting point for a conceptualization of emotion in terms of central nervous system processes. It will therefore first be appropriate to consider findings pertaining to the location of central nervous system areas associated with the activation of pleasure and unpleasure and of related states of reward and punishment.

Chapters I and II deal respectively with limbic system contributions to reactions of pleasure and unpleasure and with limbic system contributions to reticular non-specific activation. A possible relation between these psychological and physiological processes is considered in Chapter III.

Definitions

Reward mechanisms are defined as certain central nervous system processes whose excitation reinforces the maintenance and repetition of on-going conditional responses to on-going stimuli.° *Reward stimulus conditions* are external or internal conditions which innervate these central nervous system reward mechanisms.

Punishment mechanisms are defined as certain central nervous system processes, innervation of which disrupts and inhibits the maintenance and repetition of on-going conditional responses to on-going stimuli. *Punishment stimulus conditions* are external or internal conditions which innervate these central nervous system punishment mechanisms.

Pleasure is defined as the diffuse perceptual experience generally accompanying the release of reward mechanisms.

° "Conditional response" indicates "changeable response": response which is not permanently fixed in relation to the presentation of a particular stimulus. In contrast, "unconditional response" indicates "unchanging response": a response like the knee jerk which qualitatively cannot be changed in relation to the presentation of a particular stimulus.

3

Unpleasure or displeasure is defined as the diffuse perceptual experience generally accompanying the release of punishment mechanisms.

Operational Procedures for Mapping Anatomically Those Areas of the CNS Involved with Pleasure and Unpleasure, Reward and Punishment

Significant advances in scientific knowledge often depend upon the creation and development of a new instrument or procedure for observing ongoing events. An unquestionable advance in the field of neurophysiology was made when the Swiss neurophysiologist, W.R. Hess (1932), introduced a technique for electrically stimulating localized areas of the central nervous system by means of electrodes chronically implanted in active, freely moving subjects. Prior to the development of this technique, physiological investigation of the central nervous system was carried out by means of stimulation of anesthetized or immobilized subjects, or by behavioral observation of the gross effects of lesions of the brain. The chronically implanted electrode technique for the first time made it directly possible to correlate neurophysiological changes taking place within the central nervous system with psychological changes in the subject's spontaneous behavior. More specifically, the chronically implanted electrode technique has led to the development of the following procedures for the detection of those central nervous system areas whose stimulation releases reward-pleasure or punishment-unpleasure effects upon behavior.

1. *Intracranial Electrical Self-stimulation Studies Among Animals*

Olds and Milner (1954:419) introduced the technique of self-stimulation of chronically implanted electrodes in relation to the study of CNS reward mechanisms among animals. Delgado, Roberts, and Miller (1954:587) simultaneously introduced a similar technique for the study of CNS punishment mechanisms. Over a period of more than ten years, Olds (1964:22–53) has extended the use of this technique to delineate within the central nervous system those areas whose stimulation elicits reward and those areas whose stimulation elicits punishment effects. Typically, Olds employed the following procedure in these studies:

(a) Electrodes were implanted at numerous fixed locations within the central nervous system for each animal subject.

(b) Animal subjects, following recovery from electrode implantation, were individually placed in a typical behavioral testing situation employing a Skinner box with a depressable lever as described by the diagram in Figure I-1.

(c) Fine-gauge wires, spring-suspended from above, were connected to

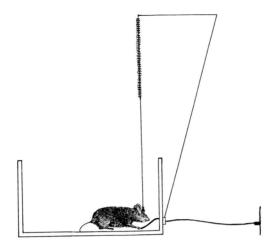

G.D.V.

Figure I-1. "Sketch of bar-pressing device by which a rat administers electric shock to its own brain." (Quoted and adapted with permission, from Olds, J.: Self stimulation of the brain. *Science, 127*:315, 1958, Fig. 1.).

the implanted electrodes which were insulated except for the bared tips and which thus permitted the administration of electrical stimulation to localized regions in the animal's brain.

(d) The animal subject was free to move and perform within the testing situation.

(e) Electrical stimulation, with carefully specified stimulus parameters, was automatically delivered to the implanted electrodes every time the animal depressed the lever.

(f) The reward or punishment effects resulting from electrical stimulation of specified areas of the brain could be assessed in terms of the rate and persistence of lever pressing.

2. Human Intracranial Electrical Stimulation Studies

Heath (1964:219–23) introduced the technique of eliciting pleasure and unpleasure by stimulating electrodes chronically implanted within the human brain. He and his group at Tulane have used this technique with chronic schizophrenic patients and were able to quote the patients' reports of feelings of pleasure and unpleasure elicited only when certain specific areas of the central nervous system were stimulated. Electrodes were implanted within carefully delineated areas of the brain of each subject. Table I reproduced from Heath (1964:221) lists typical placement areas. Electrical stimulation was applied to each electrode at specified times. The subject's emotional behavior and verbal reports were then observed and recorded.

TABLE I
ELECTRODE PLACEMENTS
(Placement in Patient No. B-12)

Site	Electrodes
L. temporal cortex	8 regular
R. temporal cortex	8 regular
L. occipital cortex	5 regular
R. occipital cortex	5 regular
L. frontal cortex	2 regular + 1 stainless steel
R. frontal cortex	3 regular
L. parietal cortex	2 regular
R. parietal cortex	2 regular
L. centromedian	1 stainless steel
R. centromedian	1 stainless steel
L. caudate	1 regular + 1 stainless steel
L. ventricle	1 regular
R. ventricle	1 regular
L. hippocampus	1 stainless steel
R. hippocampus	1 stainless steel
L. hypothalamus	1 stainless steel
R. hypothalamus	2 stainless steel
L. septal	1 stainless steel
R. septal	1 regular + 1 stainless steel
R. amygdala	1 stainless steel

As a variation of this technique in which the subject passively receives electrode stimulation under the control of the experimental examiner, Heath (ibid: 222) and his group also employed a procedure in which the subject depressed a button to self-stimulate his brain. In this way, the examiner was able to observe (a) reactions typically associated with pleasure and unpleasure—smiling, laughing, scowling, dejection, etc., (b) verbal reports of pleasure and unpleasure, and (c) the reward-maintenance and punishment-disruption effects upon the patient's button-pressing behavior.

3. *Intracranial Chemical Stimulation Studies*

Chemical substances, e.g., acetylcholine, atropine, histamine, may be introduced into specific CNS locations via cannulae (Heath, 1964:223). This technique has been used in the same way as the electrode-implantation techniques for the detection of CNS areas involved with reactions of pleasure and unpleasure.

4. *Recording Localized EEG Changes During Pleasurable and Unpleasurable Conversation*

The procedure of measuring brain electrical activity during pleasurable and unpleasurable conversation and thought has been presented in detail by Heath and Gallant (1964:83–86) who point out: "The electrode implantation methods developed at Tulane University permit recording of electrical activity from these deep systems and from the surface of the scalp simultaneously with subjective mental activity . . . The patients prepared with depth electrodes were studied psychologically while physiologic data were recorded synchronously from a large number of regions of the brain . . . we were able to correlate some types of reproducible electrical activity in specific areas of the brain with patterns of thought activity . . . The recording change could be induced through direction of the interview by the psychiatrist into specific associations."

Whereas other techniques involve stimulating the central nervous system first and subsequently observing changes of pleasure and unpleasure, the present technique involves evoking reactions of pleasure and unpleasure first and subsequently observing EEG changes.

Experimental Findings With Respect to Discovery of CNS Areas Whose Stimulation Elicits Reactions of Pleasure-Reward and Unpleasure-Punishment: the Limbic System

Studies using the above-mentioned techniques all point to the same conclusions: the cortical and subcortical points from which may be elicited reward and pleasure, punishment and unpleasure reactions, are contained

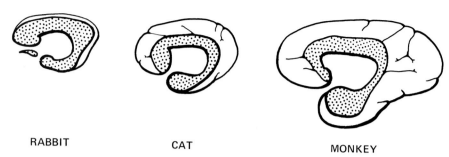

RABBIT　　　　CAT　　　　MONKEY

G.D.V.

Figure I-2. The limbic system, represented in gray, comprises most of the lower mammalian cortex. Among more highly developed species, the limbic system becomes enveloped by a neocortical mantle. (Redrawn with permission, from MacLean, P., in Wittkower, E., and Cleghorn, R., Eds.: *Recent Developments in Psychosomatic Medicine*. London: Pitman Press, 1954.)

within the *limbic system*. This section, therefore, will briefly review the anatomy of this system.

MacLean (1963:17–18) writes that the limbic system is the equivalent of the lower mammalian brain which consists of the phylogenetically old cortex and its related nuclei.* Figure I-2, reproduced from MacLean (ibid:18), illustrates how most of the cortex of the lower mammalian is found in the limbic lobe.

Additionally, the relative positions of individual components of the limbic system are presented in Figures I-3, I-4, and I-6. The diagrams suggest their relationship to the neocortex, thalamus, hypothalamus, and brainstem.

Table II lists the principal constituents of the limbic system and indicates their position within the CNS. References to the literature provide a source for more detailed information with respect to each area.

The interrelation of these upper, central, and lower limbic areas becomes clarified as one examines available information with respect to the neural pathways existing within the limbic system. The chart in Figure I-5 schematically describes prominent descending pathways. Table III lists pertinent references.

Of Note

1. The fornix connects the hippocampus with the hypothalamus. The stria terminalis connects the amygdala with the hypothalamus. The medial forebrain bundle connects the septal nuclei with the hypothalamus. Thus

---

* The prefrontal cortex most likely is a limbic system derivative which has developed at a later phylogenetic period (Nauta, 1964:405).

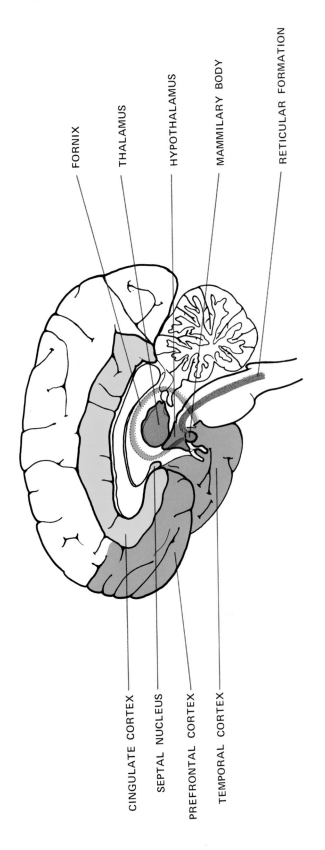

CINGULATE CORTEX

SEPTAL NUCLEUS

PREFRONTAL CORTEX

TEMPORAL CORTEX

FORNIX

THALAMUS

HYPOTHALAMUS

MAMMILARY BODY

RETICULAR FORMATION

G.D.V.

Figure I-3. The limbic system, medial sagittal view.

TABLE II
THE LIMBIC SYSTEM

Limbic System Constituent	Position Within the Limbic System	General Structure and Position Within the Central Nervous System	Reference
Reticular formation	Lower limbic	An internuncial network within the brainstem, midbrain, and thalamus; contains the tegmental reticular nuclei	French, 1960:1281–4 Brady, 1958:195, 202–3
Hypothalamus	Central limbic	Diencephalic core of the limbic system	Brady, ibid:195 House and Pansky, 1967:403–10
Septal nucleus	Upper limbic	A subcortical component of the limbic system, anterior and superior to the hypothalamus	Brady, ibid:195 Crosby, 1962:419
Amygdaloid nucleus	Upper limbic	A subcortical component of the limbic system embedded within the temporal cortex	Gloor, 1960:1395 Brady, 1958:195
Hippocampus	Upper limbic	Primitive ancient **"paleo-"** ("archi") three-layered cortex which together with the pyriform cortex forms the bulk of the cerebral hemispheres in lower vertebrates	Green, 1960:1374 Brady, 1958:195 Grossman, 1967:528
Pyriform, (Entorhinal) cortex	Upper limbic	Primitive ancient **"paleo-"** three-layered cortex lying on the ventral aspect of the temporal lobe	Brady, 1958:195 Green, 1960:1373
Cingulate cortex	Upper limbic	**"Meso-"** four to five-layered newer limbic cortex medially forming an arch above the corpus callosum	Brady, 1958:195 Kaada, 1960:1345–6 Grossman, 1967:528
Orbito-insular-temporal cortex	Upper limbic	**"Meso-"** four to five-layered limbic cortex contributing to the formation of the anterior-medial and basal cerebrum	Kaada, ibid:1346–7 Grossman, 1967:528
Prefrontal cortex	Upper limbic	Six-layered limbic **"neo-"** cortex of the anterior cerebrum	Nauta, 1964:405 Akert, 1964:377–8

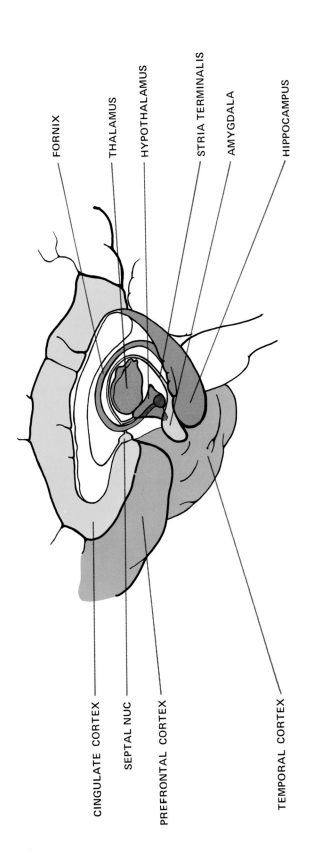

FORNIX

THALAMUS

HYPOTHALAMUS

STRIA TERMINALIS

AMYGDALA

HIPPOCAMPUS

CINGULATE CORTEX

SEPTAL NUC

PREFRONTAL CORTEX

TEMPORAL CORTEX

G.D.V.

Figure I-4. The limbic system, sagittal view.

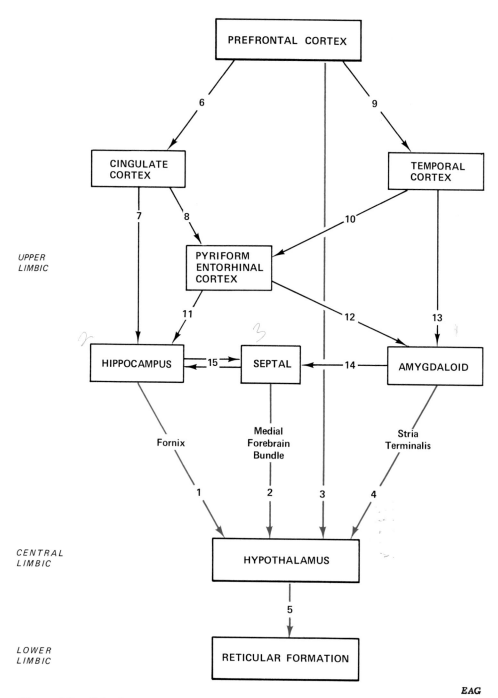

Figure I-5. All limbic roads lead to the hypothalamus and reticular formation.

TABLE III
ANATOMICAL CONNECTIONS WITHIN THE LIMBIC SYSTEM [*]

Connection		Reference
1. Hippocampus ⟶	Hypothalamus	House and Pansky, 1967:403
2. Septal Nuclei ⟶	Hypothalamus	House and Pansky, 1967:220
3. Prefrontal Cortex ⟶	Hypothalamus	Nauta, 1964:403
4. Amygdala ⟶	Hypothalamus	Ingram, 1960:964 Ruch, 1965:240
5. Hypothalamus ⟶	Reticular Formation	Ingram, 1960:964–5 House and Pansky, 1967:409 Ruch, 1965:240
6. Prefrontal Cortex ⟶	Cingulate Cortex	Nauta, 1964:397–9
7, 8. Cingulate Cortex ⟶	Hippocampus and Pyriform Cortex	Nauta, 1964:397 Green, 1960:1377
9. Prefrontal Cortex ⟶	Temporal Cortex	Nauta, 1964:399–400
10. Temporal Cortex ⟶	Pyriform Cortex	Crosby, 1962:428
11. Pyriform Cortex ⟶	Hippocampus	Nauta, 1964:397 Green, 1960:1376 Brady, 1958:196
12. Pyriform Cortex ⟶	Amygdala	Kappers, 1936:1436
13. Temporal Cortex ⟶	Amygdala	Nauta, 1964:401
14. Amygdala ⟶	Septal Nuclei	Gloor, 1960:1399
15. Septal Nuclei ⟶	Hippocampus	Kappers, 1936:1408

[*] Numbers employed in the table refer to specific tracts listed in Fig. I-5.

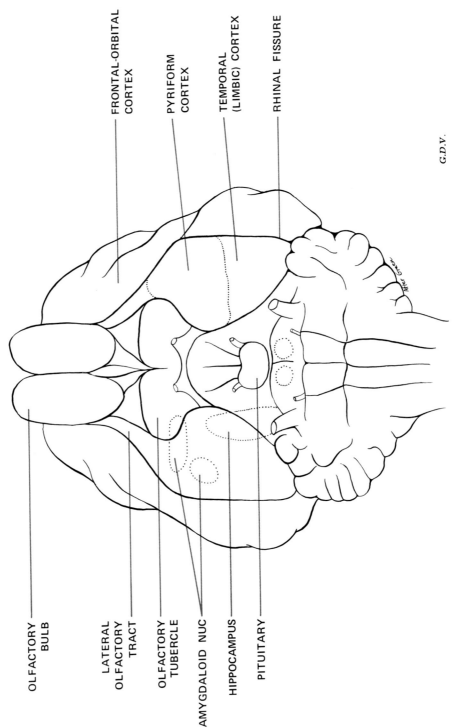

Figure I-6. The limbic system, basal view of the cat brain. (Redrawn with permission, from Green, J.: *J Comp Neurol, 108:*505, 1957.

the fornix, the stria terminalis, the medial forebrain bundle, as well as the tracts descending from the prefrontal cortex, combine to connect the upper components with the hypothalamic core of the limbic system.

2. The medial forebrain bundle* (see Olds, 1964:31–2), not only connects upper limbic nuclei such as the septal nuclei with the hypothalamus, but also courses through the hypothalamus and lower limbic system. Within the hypothalamus it becomes the lateral hypothalamic tube. Upon emerging from the hypothalamus, its fibres become distributed to nuclei enmeshed within the internuncial reticular formation.

3. The periventricular system of fibres (see Ingram, 1960:964) also connects the hypothalamus with the reticular formation of the thalamus and midbrain.

The Limbic System In Relation to
Pleasure and Reward, Unpleasure and Punishment

Table IV summarizes the results of experimental studies delineating CNS loci whose functions are related to pleasure and reward, unpleasure and punishment.

The presentation of these findings in Table IV becomes more meaningful as one examines some of the details reported from the literature.

Heath's studies (1964: 224–5) illustrate the extent of these human reactions to self-stimulation of chronically implanted electrodes: "With septal stimulation the patients brightened . . . Expressions of anguish, self-condemnation and despair changed precipitously to expressions of *optimism* and elaboration of pleasant experiences, past and anticipated . . . Subjects were not informed when stimuli were applied. When questioned concerning changes in mental content, they were generally at a loss to explain them. For example, one patient on the verge of tears described his father's near fatal illness and condemned himself as somehow responsible," but following stimulation "he immediately terminated this conversation and within 15 seconds exhibited a broad grin as he discussed plans to date and seduce a girl friend. When asked why he had changed the conversation so abruptly, he replied that the plans concerning the girl suddenly came to him. This phenomenon was repeated several times in the patient. Stimulation was administered . . . when he was describing a depressive state, and almost instantly he became gay. Another severely agitated and depressed subject whose verbalization expressed self-condemnation and hopelessness (a condition that had prevailed for over 2 years), smiled broadly and related a sexual experience of his youth within one minute after onset of septal stimulation. Only rarely was there objective evidence of sexual arousal." The

---

* Among higher vertebrates a system of fibres corresponding to the medial forebrain bundle of amphibia (P. Yakovlev, personal communication).

TABLE IV
STIMULATION OF THE LIMBIC SYSTEM:
PLEASURE, REWARD, UNPLEASURE AND PUNISHMENT EFFECTS

Area Studied	Reference	Experimental Technique	Results
1. UPPER LIMBIC AREAS **Septal nuclei**	Olds, 1958:246	Animal intracranial self-stimulation	**Reward** associated with **septal** self-stimulation
	Olds, 1964:26	Animal intracranial self-stimulation	**Reward** associated with **septal** self-stimulation
	Heath, 1964:224	Human intracranial passive stimulation; subjects' report of emotional responses	**Pleasure** associated with **septal** stimulation
	Heath, ibid:233,235	Human intracranial chemical stimulation with acetylcholine; observation of local EEG changes during report of emotional experience	**Pleasure** associated with chemical stimulation of the **septal** nuclei and with EEG changes in the **septal** nuclei
Amygdaloid nuclei	Olds, 1958:246	Animal intracranial self-stimulation	**Reward** associated with **amygdaloid** self-stimulation
	Olds, 1964:26	Animal intracranial self-stimulation	**Reward** associated with **amygdaloid** self-stimulation
	Heath, 1964:228–9, incl. Table 2	Human intracranial self-stimulation	**Reward** and **pleasure** associated with **amygdaloid** self-stimulation
Cingulate cortex	Olds, 1958:248		

Structure	Reference	Method	Finding
			self-stimulation
	Heath and Gallant, 1964:87	Localized EEG changes (during conversation of pleasurable memories)	**Pleasure** reported accompanying EEG changes in the **hippocampus**
2. HYPOTHALAMUS			
Lat. hypothalamic tube: medial forebrain bundle	Olds, 1958:246	Animal intracranial self-stimulation	**Reward** associated with **hypothalamic** self-stimulation
	Olds, 1964:26	Animal intracranial self-stimulation	**Reward** associated with **hypothalamic** self-stimulation
	Heath, 1964:226	Human intracranial passive stimulation with subjects' report of perceptual response	**Pleasure** "good feeling" associated with **hypothalamic** stimulation
3. RETICULAR FORMATION Thalamic reticulum:	Bishop, Elder, and Heath, 1964:70	Human intracranial self-stimulation	**Reward** associated with **reticular formation** self-stimulation
	Heath, 1964:228	Human intracranial self-stimulation	**Reward** associated with **reticular formation** self-stimulation
Midbrain reticular formation: medial forebrain bundle terminating in midbrain tegmentum	Heath, 1964:228, Table 2	Human intracranial self-stimulation	**Pleasure** associated with tegmental **reticular formation** self-stimulation
	Heath, 1964:224	Human, intracranial passive stimulation	**Reward** associated with tegmental **reticular formation** stimulation

TABLE IV – (Continued)

Area Studied	Reference	Experimental Technique	Results
1. UPPER LIMBIC AREAS **Hippocampus**	Heath, 1964:227	Human intracranial self-stimulation	**Mild punishment** accompanying **hippocampal** self-stimulation
	Heath and Gallant, 1964:96	Local EEG changes during reporting of emotional experiences	**Unpleasure** "intensely painful" emotional experience accompanied by EEG changes in the **hippocampus**
	Heath, 1964:226	Human intracranial passive stimulation	**Unpleasure,** pronounced anxiety, accompanying **hippocampal** stimulation
	Heath, ibid:235 incl. Fig. 8	Localized intracranial administration of acetylcholine in human subjects; recording of localized EEG changes during report of emotional experience	**Unpleasure,** (rage, fear, or depression) accompanied by EEG changes in the **hippocampus**
Amygdaloid nuclei	Heath and Gallant, 1964:96	Human local EEG changes during reporting of emotional experiences	**Unpleasure** "intensely painful" emotional experience accompanied by **amygdala** EEG changes
	Heath, 1964:235, Fig. 8	Human local EEG changes during reporting of emotional experiences	**Unpleasure** "feelings of despair" accompanied by **amygdala** EEG changes
Septal nuclei	Heath and Gallant, 1964:90	Human local EEG changes during	**Unpleasure** intense anger accompanied by

		self-stimulation	accompanying stimulation of **hypothalamic** periventricular system
hypothalamus	Olds, 1958:247	Animal intracranial self-stimulation	**Punishment** accompanying self-stimulation of **hypothalamus**
Rostral hypothalamus	Heath, 1964:226	Human intracranial passive stimulation	**Unpleasure** "discomfort" associated with visceral disturbances accompanying stimulation of **hypothalamus**
3. RETICULAR FORMATION **Dorsal aspects of midbrain tegmentum**	Olds, 1964:32, Fig. 6	Animal intracranial self-stimulation	**Punishment** accompanying stimulation of dorsal tegmental **reticular formation** of midbrain
Midline tegmentum of reticular formation	Heath, 1964,226, 227	Human intracranial passive stimulation	**Unpleasure** (rage or fear and pain) accompanying stimulation of midline tegmentum of **reticular formation**

author went on to speak of other studies in which "Striking and immediate relief from intractable physical pain was consistently obtained with stimulation . . . of 3 patients with advanced carcinoma, 2 with metastases from primary breast carcinoma to bone, and 1 with carcinoma of the cervix and extensive local proliferation. The patients were stimulated at intervals ranging from twice a day to once every 3 days over periods of 3 weeks to 8 months. Stimulation . . . immediately relieved the intense physical pain and anguish, and the patients relaxed in comfort and pleasure."

The pleasure and unpleasure, reward and punishment effects obtained by human self-stimulation of the limbic system are exemplified by another of Heath's reports of studies with schizophrenic patients (ibid:227): Patient No. B-7 pressed the septal button almost exclusively (reward effects). On the other hand, when he pressed the button associated with the mesencephalic tegmentum of the reticular formation, "he complained of intense discomfort, looked fearful and requested that the stimulus to the mesencephalic tegmentum not be repeated although it induced alerting. To make certain that the region was not stimulated again" (punishment effect), "he ingeniously modified a hairpin to fit under the button . . . so it could not be depressed. The patient found stimulation to the hippocampus to be mildly aversive" (unpleasure-punishment effects) "whereas stimulation to the septal region was most rewarding and caused alerting. When asked why he pressed the septal button with such frequency, the patient said the feeling was 'good' . . . ." (pleasurable).

EEG changes localized within the limbic system have occurred concomitantly with the subject's reports of pleasurable and unpleasurable experiences. A quotation from Heath and Gallant (1964:87) illustrates such experimental findings: "In Patient A-10, for example, high spindling began in the hippocampus when he recalled a television program on juvenile delinquency that he had seen the previous evening and that recalled extremely disturbing boyhood memories. This electrical activity persisted until he was given a simple mathematical problem. As he began to calculate, the spindling stopped. . . . On another occasion, an interview with the same patient was directed toward pleasurable associations. The subject was asked if at any time in his life he had experienced intensely good feelings. Promptly high amplitude 14 per second hippocampal activity reappeared as he recalled a rare sense of well-being and success. . . ." And in another case, Heath (1964:236–8) writes of EEG changes within the septal region taking place at the same time that his patient "smiled and became euphoric."

An inquiry into the nature of the non-specific activating systems will lead to a consideration of the intriguing question of what processes possibly may account for these upper limbic, hypothalamic and reticular contributions to states of pleasure and unpleasure.

Chapter II

Upper Limbic-Hypothalamic-Reticular Contributions to Non-Specific Activation

The Concepts of "Specificity" and "Non-specificity"

S *pecificity* refers to *demarcated change* with respect to on-going conditions. Specificity in relation to the distribution of sensory impulses within the central nervous system refers to the projection of impulses from a highly demarcated, localized point of a sensory receptor surface (e.g., of the retina, cochlea, or skin) to a highly demarcated, localized point within the thalamus or cortex (e.g., see Fig. IV-3.)

Conversely *non-specificity* refers to a *paucity of demarcated change* and to a high degree of constancy. Non-specificity in relation to the distribution of sensory impulses within the central nervous system refers to a projection of impulses upon the thalamus or cerebral cortex, a projection which involves a paucity of demarcated change from one point to another and one area to another.

Ascending Reticular Non-specfic Irradiations to the Neocortex and Paleocortex

Lorente de Nó (1938:299) first described the presence of an ascending diffuse network of fibres which becomes distributed throughout the cerebral cortex. Morison and Dempsey (1942:292) drew attention to two contrasting sensory systems between thalamus and cortex: "a well-known specific projection system with a more or less point-to-point arrangement; a secondary non-specific system with diffuse connections." Subsequent experimental evidence (see Nauta, 1958:3–4, 22–3) has indicated that the reticular formation of the hindbrain, midbrain, and thalamus, and their irradiations to the cerebral cortex, form the core of this ascending non-specific projection system. The reticular formation by definition refers to the primi-

21

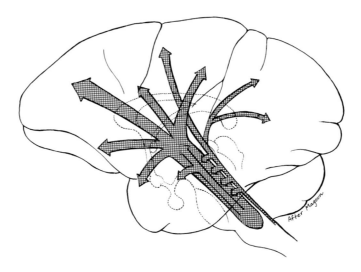

G.D.V.

Figure II-1. The ascending reticular non-specific projection system. (Redrawn with permission, from Magoun, H.W.: The ascending reticular system and wakefulness. In Delafresnaye, J., Ed.: *Brain Mechanism and Consciousness*. Oxford: Blackwell Press, 1954.)

tively organized, lace-like network which is neither sensory nor motor but forms an internuncial system. Figure II-1 depicts the non-specific reticular projection system. Figure II-2 is based upon experimental findings which have been summarized by Jasper (1960:1307–19) and by French (1960: 1282–7). It includes reference to the finding that non-specific irradiations from the midbrain reticular formation reach the neocortex via two routes, one a direct route which bypasses the thalamus, the other an indirect route via the medial reticular areas of the thalamus.

The sensory input into the non-specific reticular system derives from all sensory modalities and all body sectors. French (ibid:1284) notes: A single electrode placed within the reticular formation can record responses from stimuli applied to a variety of conductor or receptor systems, for example, from stimulation of the sciatic, the sympathetic, and the radial nerves as well as from an audible click. In other words, impulses from all sensory receptors are funneled into the internuncial reticulum of the midbrain and thalamus (Fig. II-2) where fusion of these impulses takes place before they are distributed diffusely throughout the cortex. The convergence of sensory impulses upon the internuncial reticulum of the midbrain and thalamus and their diffuse distribution to the cerebral cortex form a process comparable to the preparation of a Hawaiian punch which becomes distributed to surrounding guests. In a Hawaiian punch preparation, individual specific fruit juices are mixed together and then distributed equally in homogenized

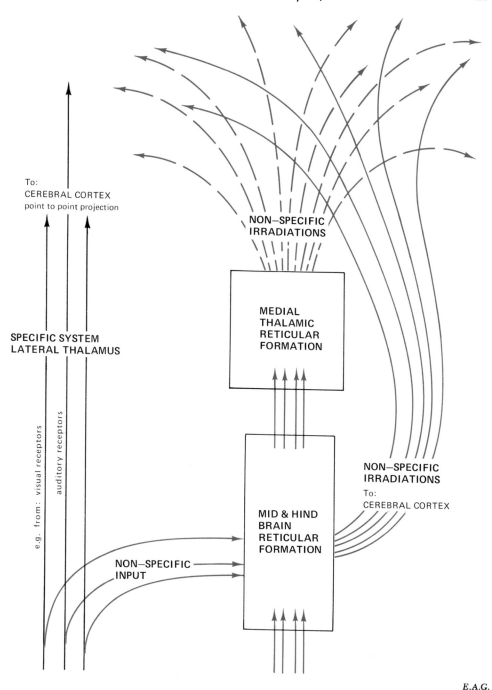

Figure II-2. Ascending reticular non-specific irradiations to the cortex.

form to each guest. Likewise, within the reticular formation there occurs *fusion* of input and sameness of output providing a basis for the non-specific, non-demarcated character of the ascending non-specific systems of the internuncial reticulum.

Figure II-2 indicates conversely that the organization of the specific ascending sensory systems involves neither fusion of sensory impulses nor a diffuse distribution throughout the cerebral cortex, but rather demarcated change or separateness of ascending sensory pathways. It also draws attention to the experimental findings that the specific ascending sensory systems are associated with the lateral portions of the thalamus, whereas the non-specific systems are associated with the medial reticular portions of the thalamus (see Pribram, 1960:1326, Fig. 2 and notation; Jasper, 1960:1314, Fig. 6).

The Ascending Reticular Non-specific Activating System

The midbrain and thalamic reticular non-specific irradiations to the cerebral cortex form the anatomical core of what has come to be known as the reticular non-specific activating system. This concept was formally introduced by Moruzzi and Magoun (1949:471) who employed EEG techniques to measure the diffuse cortical effects arising from the stimulation of the brainstem reticular formation.

The processes of the ascending specific and non-specific systems have been shown to react synergistically within the thalamus and cerebral cortex, a function of the overlapping projections of the two systems (Jasper, 1960: 1315). This neuroanatomical interrelationship provides a basis whereby the processes of non-specific activation may potentiate, or inhibit, specifically innervated cortical perceptual and motor processes. The level of ascending reticular non-specific activation, as reflected by the electroencephalogram, correlates closely with degrees of perceptual consciousness and wakeful behavior (Magoun, 1958:25). Conscious perception is understood to be a function of non-specific potentiation of specific sensory engrams or images; wakeful behavior, a function of non-specific potentiation of specific motor engrams. The synergy of the specific and non-specific systems may be compared to the interaction of the keyboard and pedal mechanisms of a musical organ. The production of an overt tone during the depression of a specific note of the keyboard is dependent upon the non-specific diffuse effects that are derived from pumping the organ pedal. Non-specific processes are essential for overt effects in the case of both the musical organ and the perceptual processes of the central nervous system: without non-specific potentiation neither does a specific organ tone become amplified nor a specific perception become conscious (Lindsley, 1960:1559).

Although both the midbrain and thalamic reticular systems contribute to these non-specific processes, each system is characterized by certain significant differences.

Characteristics of Midbrain Reticular Non-specific Activation

Midbrain reticular activation is referred to in the literature as tonic (Jasper, 1960: 1318). Characterized by extreme degrees of non-specificity it demonstrates:

1. Deficiency in its capacity to respond differentially to changes in *stimulus spatial distribution*. According to this concept, demarcated change in the distribution of stimulation from the hands to the feet (total magnitude of stimulation a constant) does not result in a corresponding change in the distribution of non-specific activation within the thalamus or cerebral cortex.

2. Deficiency in its capacity to respond differentially to demarcated changes in *stimulus temporal distribution*. The temporal aspects of tonic non-specific activation may hypothetically be represented by the schematic diagram in Figure II-3.

Arduini (1963: 187) concludes: "The attribute 'tonic' . . . implies a non-transient condition . . . It can be said that . . . an activity is tonic when it

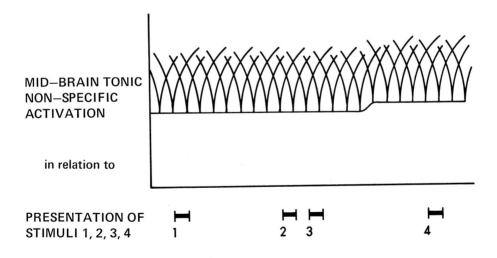

MID–BRAIN TONIC NON–SPECIFIC ACTIVATION

in relation to

PRESENTATION OF STIMULI 1, 2, 3, 4

1   2   3   4

E.A.G.

Figure II-3. Midbrain tonic non-specific activation demonstrates a deficient capacity to reflect stimulus temporal patterns.

does not have a time relationship with any particular event." This extreme degree of spatial and temporal non-specificity is presumably a function of the marked diffuseness both of the midbrain reticular cytoarchitecture (the "Hawaiian punch" mixing bowl) and of its irradiations to the cerebral cortex.

3. Definite capacity to respond differentially to *changes in stimulus intensity.* Moruzzi (1956: 272) has shown that reticular discharge is characterized by a number of different resting rhythms, i.e., by (a) low frequencies 2–5/sec., (b) frequencies sustained at 50–100/sec., and (c) spike outbursts of 50–70/sec. These rhythms may be shifted as the result of a general increase in stimulus intensity irrespective of receptor sites. Lindsley (1960:1554) points out that such changes of reticular rhythm in turn determine parallel changes in the level of arousal of consciousness and wakefulness from subwaking states, through normal waking activity, to states of extreme excitement (see Table VIII).

4. A special capacity for *adaptation.* Adaptation involves a reduction in the number of active neuronal units during continued repetition of the same stimulus (Dell: 1963, 82–3). Jasper (1958: 55–6) points out that an initial startling stimulus is always far more effective than the repetition of the same stimulus in influencing levels of midbrain tonic non-specific activation.

Characteristics of Thalamic Reticular
Non-specific Activation

Thalamic reticular activation is referred to in the literature (Jasper, 1960: 1318) as phasic. It is characterized basically by temporal and spatial non-specificity. Additionally it demonstrates:

1. Some minimal capacity to respond differentially to changes in *stimulus temporal distribution.* According to Jasper (ibid:1318) thalamic phasic non-specific activation is of rapid onset and brief duration, i.e., onset and termination of stimuli result in rapid onset and termination of thalamic phasic non-specific activation (Fig. II-4). This capacity contrasts with the incapacity of midbrain tonic non-specific activation to reflect temporal patterns of stimulation (see Fig. II-3). Lindsley (1960: 1562) suggests that the tonic midbrain activating system determines longer-lasting general states of alertness while the phasic thalamic activating system modulates these states on a shorter and more variable temporal scale.

2. Some capacity to respond differentially to changes in the *modality of stimulation.* Input into the thalamic reticulum from the auditory sensory receptors contributes not only to the general level of non-specific activation of the total cortex but in particular to the non-specific activation of the auditory cortex. Thalamic reticular potentiation of the specific engrams within the auditory cortex are depicted in Figure II-5 as momentarily

ONSET AND
TERMINATION OF
THALAMIC PHASIC
NON—SPECIFIC
ACTIVATION

in relation to

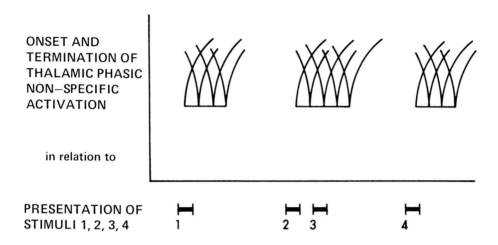

PRESENTATION OF
STIMULI 1, 2, 3, 4

E.A.G.

Figure II-4. Thalamic phasic non-specific activation demonstrates some capacity to reflect stimulus temporal patterns.

greater than within the visual cortex. The reader may picture the accentuation of thalamic non-specific activation changing from one lobe of the cerebral cortex to another.

Jasper (1958: 59) suggests that this topographical distribution of thalamic phasic non-specific activation may provide a neurophysiological basis for the direction of attention and arousal.

3. A capacity for *recruitment*. Recruitment implies that "more and more units, or increments to the field of activity, have been brought into synchrony" during an initial change in stimulus presentation (Lindsley, 1960: 1562). Dempsey and Morison's (1942: 293) experimental studies have shown that the first three or four shocks to the reticular areas of the thalamus produce a gradually increasing magnitude or recruitment of non-specific response. Repeated stimulation beyond this point is followed by a state of total activation (ibid:1562). This capacity of the thalamic phasic non-specific activating system for recruitment complements the capacity of the midbrain tonic non-specific activating system for adaptation.

4. Some capacity to produce *qualitative diffuse sensory experience*. This conclusion derives from the findings that the processes of the non-specific reticular areas of the thalamus contribute to the production of diffuse pleasurable sensation and pain (Head, 1920: 555-7, 559-60; Bowsher, 1957: 606-22).

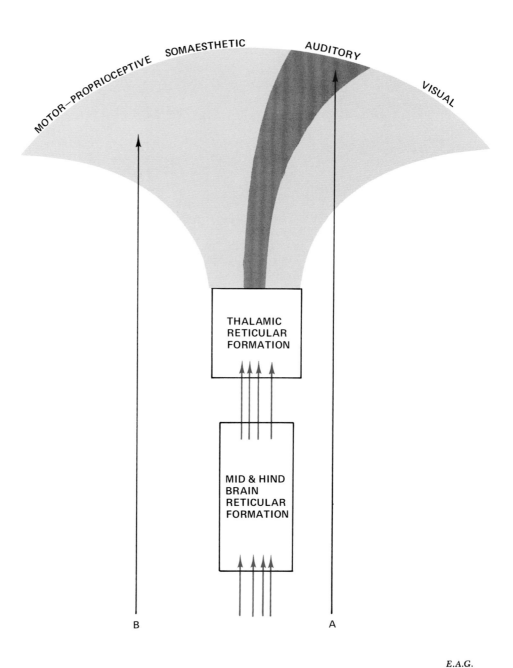

E.A.G.

Figure II-5. Thalamic reticular non-specific activation of the cortex with an accentuated distribution to the auditory cortex.

TABLE V
DIFFERENTIATING CHARACTERISTICS OF
THE MIDBRAIN AND THALAMIC NON-SPECIFIC ACTIVATING SYSTEMS

	Nomenclature	Neuroanatomy	Neurophysiological Functions	Psychological Effects upon Consciousness and Wakefulness
MIDBRAIN RETICULAR NON-SPECIFIC ACTIVATION	Tonic	Completely diffuse irradiations	Deficiency in its capacity to respond differentially to changes in the temporal or spatial distribution of stimuli; some capacity to respond differentially to changes in total stimulus intensity; prevalence of adaptation effects	Quantitative arousal of sensory perceptions and of motor wakefulness for prolonged periods of time
THALAMIC RETICULAR NON-SPECIFIC ACTIVATION	Phasic	Highly diffuse irradiations	Some capacity to respond differentially to changes in temporal distribution of stimuli and to changes in the modality of stimulation, a basis for localized variations in the levels of non-specific activation; prevalence of recruitment effects	Momentary changes in the quantitative arousal of sensory perception and motor wakefulness; localized attention; arousal of diffuse qualitative experience such as pain

Table V summarizes these differences in the characteristics of tonic midbrain and phasic thalamic non-specific activation.

Extrinsic and Intrinsic Components of the
Reticular Non-specific Activating Systems:
Anatomical Considerations

"Extrinsic" refers to a predominance of neural pathways directly projecting to or from the periphery of the nervous system. Extrinsic pathways may form synapses within a consecutive number of areas: for example, spinal cord, thalamus, and cortex, but by definition are *not interrupted by internal neural circuits.* Conversely, "intrinsic" refers to the predominance of *internal circuits* whose reverberatory processes make possible prolongation of effects (see Rose and Woolsey, 1949:391–404).

The schematic diagram in Figure II-6 illustrates the definition of extrinsic, A, versus intrinsic, B, contributions to the non-specific reticular formation.

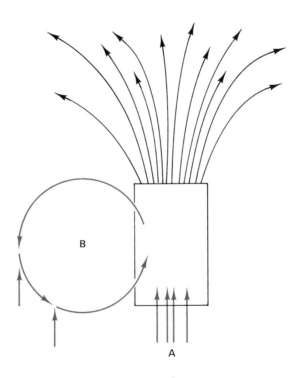

E.A.G.

Figure II-6. Extrinsic, A, versus intrinsic, B, contributions to non-specific activation.

Hypothalamic and Upper Limbic Contributions to the Reticular Non-specific Activating System

The intrinsic input into the non-specific activating system derives in great part from the hypothalamus and upper limbic areas.

Ranson and Magoun wrote in 1939 (see Lindsley, 1960:1558): "In the hypothalamus and particularly in the posterior part of the lateral hypothalamus is located a mechanism which when activated excites the entire organism . . . It is probable that the active hypothalamus not only discharges downward through the brain-stem, spinal cord and peripheral nervous system into the body, but also upward into the thalamus and cerebral cortex." This diffuse cortical excitation which follows direct stimulation of the posterior hypothalamus was observed by Gellhorn to be of the same nature as that associated with stimulation of the brain-stem reticular activating system (ibid:1558–61).

Electrode stimulation of upper limbic areas also results in non-specific activation of the cerebral cortex. Kaada (1960 : 1362) refers to a substantial number of experimental studies which indicate that stimulation of the hippocampus, the amygdala, the cingulate cortex and limbic frontal and temporal cortices, all elicit such non-specific arousal reactions.

Anatomical Bases for Hypothalamic and Upper Limbic Contributions to Ascending Non-specific Activation

Anatomical evidence suggests that the hypothalamus, upper limbic areas, and the reticular formation of the midbrain and thalamus contribute to non-specific activation via a lesser and a greater system of limbic circuits.

Table VI lists references from the experimental literature which indicate the presence of various tracts connecting the reticular formation with the hypothalamus and the hypothalamus with the reticular formation. These tracts contribute to the formation of lesser hypothalamic-reticular (h-r) circuits as schematically represented in Figure II-7.

Table VII lists tracts connecting the reticular formation, the medial-dorsal nucleus of the thalamus, the upper limbic areas, and the hypothalamus. These tracts contribute to the formation of greater upper limbic-hypothalamic-reticular (u-h-r) circuits. The diagram in Figure II-8 schematizes these findings.

The discharge of these u-h-r circuits into the reticular formation provides a most likely basis whereby the processes of individual upper limbic, hypothalamic and reticular areas contribute to ascending non-specific cortical activation. The diagram in Figure II-9 presents a condensed schematization of these relationships.

TABLE VI
LESSER H-R CIRCUITS

Connection		Reference
1. Hypothalamus	⟶ Reticular Formation and Reticular Nuc of Midbrain and Thalamus	Crosby, Humphrey, and Lauer, 1962:249 House and Pansky, 1967:409–10 Ingram, 1960:965
2. Reticular Nuc of Thalamus	⟶ Medial-Dorsal Nuc of Thalamus	Crosby, Humphrey, and Lauer, 1962:300 House and Pansky, 1967:435–6
3. Medial-Dorsal Nuc of Thalamus	⟶ Hypothalamus	Crosby, Humphrey, and Lauer, 1962:301 House and Pansky, 1967:436,403,410 Fig. 21-4

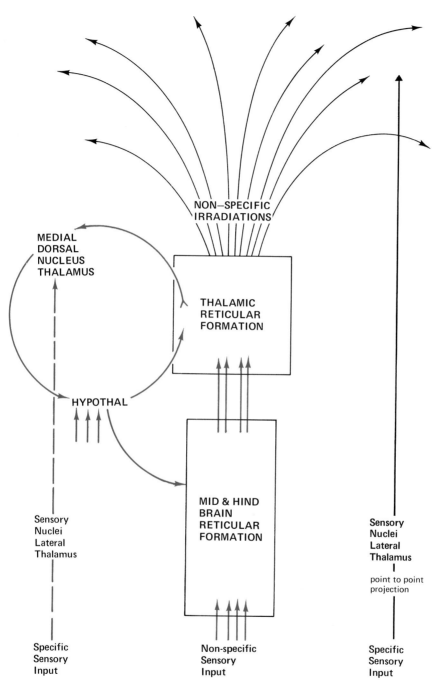

Figure II-7. The lesser h-r circuits.

TABLE VII
GREATER U-H-R CIRCUITS

Connection		Reference
1. Upper Limbic Areas ⟶	Hypothalamus	See Table III
2. Hypothalamus ⟶	Reticular Formation and Reticular Nuc of Midbrain and Thalamus	See Table VI
3. Reticular Nuc ⟶	Medial-Dorsal and Anterior Nuc of Thalamus	Crosby, 1962:300 House and Pansky, 1967:435—6
4. Medial-Dorsal, Anterior, and Reticular Nuc of Thalamus ⟶	Upper Limbic Areas	Akert, 1964:393—4 Nauta, 1964:400—1, Fig. 19.2 Crosby, Humphrey, and Lauer, 1962:30? House and Pansky, 1967:434—5 Yakovlev, 1966:83—4

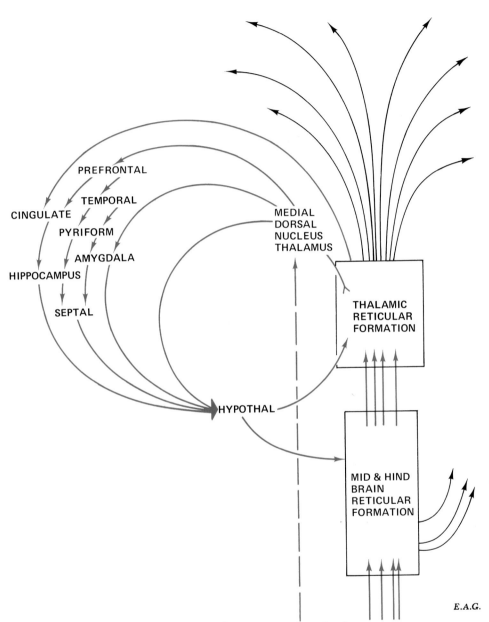

Figure II-8. The greater u-h-r circuits.

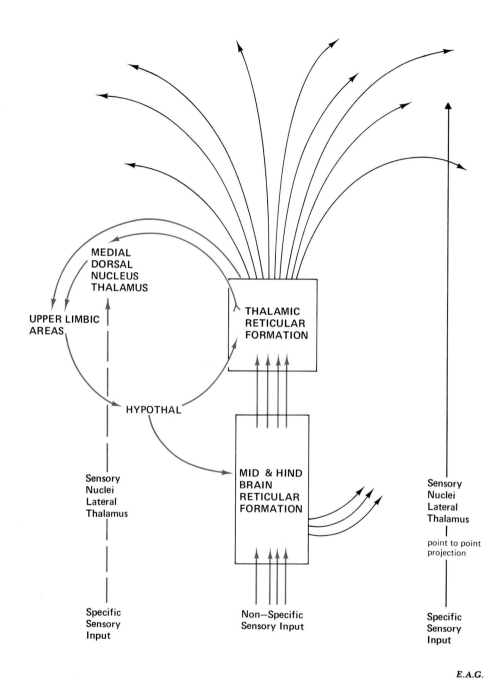

Figure II-9. The greater u-h-r circuits, condensed schematization.

The following sections will focus upon the respective roles of the hypothalamus and upper limbic areas in relation to non-specific activation.

Hypothalamic Contributions to Non-specific Activation: Neurophysiological Considerations

Hypothalamic Contributions to Intrinsic Reverberating Processes

The diagram in Figure II-7 illustrates how the association of the hypothalamus with the midbrain and thalamic reticular formation makes possible the establishment of intrinsic reverberating circuits. Such h-r circuits are in a position to be set in motion by extrinsic impulses reaching the reticular formation. They provide a neuroanatomical basis for the maintenance of a reverberating supply of impulses to reticular non-specific activation even during a momentary reduction or deficiency of extrinsic input.

The Hypothalamic Sensory Receptors

Strom (1960:1188) concludes that stimulation of the sensory receptors of the hypothalamus* by thermal changes within the bloodstream modulates the intrinsic hypothalamic input into the reticular non-specific activating system. Presumably not only thermal but also metabolic and endocrine conditions within the bloodstream provide a continually changing stimulus input into the h-r circuits (Urquhart, 1971:227, Fig. 19) which discharge via ascending non-specific activation. Thus, it is proposed that the intrinsic h-r circuits may provide for sustained contributions to non-specific activation via (1) their reverberatory processes and (2) an input from changing conditions within the bloodstream.

Upper Limbic Contributions to Ascending Non-specific Activation: Neurophysiological Considerations

The role played by upper limbic areas in relation to u-h-r circuit contributions to non-specific activation may be shown to be a function of (1) the formation of upper limbic sensory engrams, and (2) the conditional associations of such engrams with hypothalamic reactions.

Sensory Functions

Experimental and clinical investigation indicates that the upper limbic areas are associated with sensory as well as with motor functions:†

The Hippocampal Cortex   Stimulation of electrodes chronically implanted within the hippocampus was found to elicit hallucinations (Pampiglione and Falconer, 1960:1393) in patients who were were being treated for temporal lobe epilepsy. The clinical phenomena ranged from "peculiar sen-

---

* Sensory receptors embedded within the hypothalamic vasculature.
† Upper limbic motor functions are considered in Chapter IV.

sations" to complex hallucinations. Additionally, Adey's (1962:591–602) experimental studies have shown that the hippocampus is a "prime site of action" for drugs eliciting hallucination.

Amygdaloid Nuclei Electrode stimulation of the amygdala (among 46 patients who were about to undergo temporal lobe surgery for the relief of temporal lobe seizures) in nineteen cases elicited sensory-motor responses of the mouth, throat, and abdomen; in eighteen cases, somatic feelings or sensations in the head, body, and extremities; and in four, psychical hallucinations and illusions (Jasper and Rasmussen, 1958:319).

The Temporal Limbic Cortex Penfield and Perot (1963:596–695) report that in forty patients, lesions of the limbic portions of the temporal lobe were correlated with visual and auditory hallucinations. Complex sensory imagery was able to be directly evoked when specific loci within these areas were electrically stimulated. These findings indicate that the limbic temporal cortex is involved either directly or indirectly with sensory representation.

A question arises as to what ascending pathways mediate the formation and innervation of these upper limbic sensory processes. Figure II-10 refers to pertinent experimental data. Contributions from the visual, auditory, and somaesthetic areas of the neocortex are considered in Chapter XII.

The diagram in Figure II-11 illustrates the relatively specific projections from the medial-dorsal nucleus of the thalamus to the upper limbic orbito-frontal granular cortex.

Upper Limbic Sensory Processes in Relation to Conditioning of Hypothalamic Reactions

Neurological evidence indicates that upper limbic sensory processes may become conditioned to elicit certain hypothalamic and midbrain reticular reactions. Extirpation of the amygdaloid or the prefrontal cortex, for example, results in marked loss of central nervous system capacity for conditioning of hypothalamic-reticular fear reactions (Brady, 1958:213–14). Since upper limbic sensory engrams may be conditioned to elicit hypothalamic and reticular reactions, then it is proposed they may be conditioned to elicit hypothalamic facilitatory and inhibitory reactions pertaining to non-specific activation. This formulation is consistent with the experimental findings that (1) upper limbic functions affect non-specific activation (see Kaada, 1960:1362), and (2) non-specific activation reactions may be conditioned (Jasper, 1958:57). Upper limbic reverberatory processes of the u-h-r circuits could easily provide a basis for the prolongation of these effects.

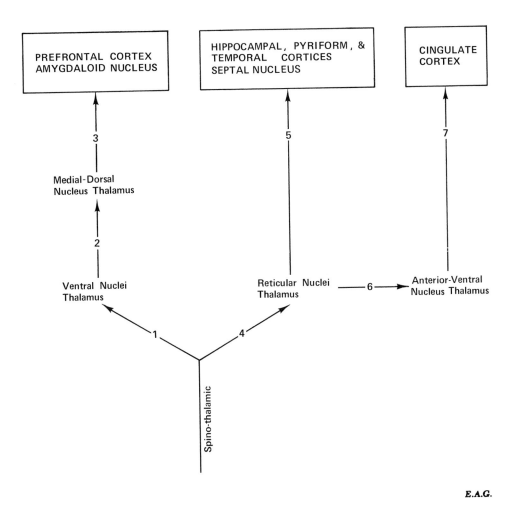

Figure II-10. Sensory paths to the upper limbic areas.

Figure II-10 references:

1, 2. Ruch, 1965:331, Fig. 12.
  3. Nauta, 1964:400–1, Fig. 19.2; Akert, 1964:393.
  4. House and Pansky, 1967:431.
  5.°Yakovlev, 1966:83–4; see Pribram, 1960:1325, Fig. 1 (re insular-temporal cortex); Brady, 1958:196.
  6. Crosby, 1962:298.
  7. Yakovlev, Locke, and Angevine, 1966:84; Walker, 1966:5.

° There has also been evidence presented more recently by P. MacLean and G. Creswell (1970:278) that sensory impulses are projected from the lateral geniculate and pulvinar nuclei of the thalamus to the hippocampal cortex.

PREFRONTAL
CORTEX

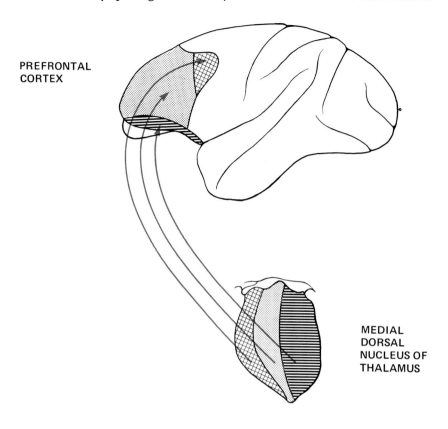

MEDIAL
DORSAL
NUCLEUS OF
THALAMUS

G.D.V.

Figure II-11. Sensory paths from the medial-dorsal nucleus of the thalamus to the prefrontal cortex. (Redrawn with permission, from Akert, K., in Warren, J., and Akert, K., Eds.: *The Frontal Granular Cortex and Behavior.* New York: McGraw-Hill, 1964, p. 393).

In summary, stimulus input into the non-specific activating systems appears to be of three types: (1) an unconditional non-specific input into the reticular formation from all sensory receptors, (2) an unconditional specific input into the hypothalamus from physical and chemical changes within the bloodstream and (3) a conditional input into the upper limbic areas from the sensory receptors. The formulation has been proposed that upper limbic sensory engrams may become established and associated with hypothalamic facilitatory or inhibitory effects upon non-specific activation.

Chapter III

An Upper Limbic-Hypothalamic-Reticular Non-specific Activation Theory of Pleasure and Unpleasure

Pleasure and Unpleasure in Relation to Intrinsic Contributions to Non-specific Activation

If u-h-r circuit stimulation elicits physiological changes with respect to reticular non-specific activation and elicits psychological changes pertaining to pleasure and unpleasure, there arises the possibility that *certain u-h-r circuit contributions to reticular non-specific activation would be the physiological equivalent of the psychological reactions of pleasure and unpleasure.* A tentative assumption that pleasure and unpleasure are functions of certain unique temporal patterns of phasic reticular non-specific activation offers a neurophysiological explanation for the differences between u-h-r contributions to arousal and to pleasure and unpleasure. According to this proposal, pleasure and unpleasure are diffuse perceptual reactions which are functions of unique patterns of activity of a reticular multisynaptic network in the vicinity of the medial thalamus. This formulation parallels Hebb's (1949:184–5) and Noordenbos' (1966:250–3) respective conclusions that pain, also a diffuse perceptual reaction, is a function of some peculiarity in the patterning of thalamic activity and is a dervative of the processes of a reticular multisynaptic network rather than of a specific nucleus or tract (see also Kruger, 1966:76). Unpleasure and pain then would be equivalent in that both are functions of particular patterns of activity associated with the non-specific multisynaptic activation processes of the thalamic reticulum (Bowsher, 1957:618–19). They would be differentiable on the basis of an extrinsic versus an intrinsic reticular input. Pain, as a sensation, most likely involves an input into the reticular formation derived from the peripheral receptors and from the slow frequency A-delta and C fibre tracts (see Sweet, 1959:469); while unpleasure, as an internal "feeling" which can persist independently of external pain stimulation, would involve an input from the reverberatory

TABLE VIII
PSYCHOLOGICAL STATES AND THEIR RELATION TO EEG
CORRELATES OF NON-SPECIFIC ACTIVATION

Psychological Manifestations in Terms of Level of Emotional Excitation	Neurophysiological Changes with Respect to Levels of Non-specific Activation Measured by EEG Recordings
Strong excited emotion: fear, rage, anxiety	Fast frequencies, desynchronized
Alert attentiveness	Mainly fast waves, partially synchronized
Relaxed wakefulness	Synchronized
Drowsiness	Occasional slow waves
Light sleep	Slow waves
Deep sleep	Very slow waves
Coma	Large slow waves
Death	Gradual and permanent disappearance of all electrical activity

Adapted with permission from Lindsley, D., Psychological phenomena and the electroencephalogram. *Electroencephalog Clin Neurophysiol,* 1952, 4:443–456; 445 Table I.

u-h-r system circuits.[*] This non-specific activation theory of pleasure and unpleasure is not original. It reflects Cannon's *thalamic* theory, Lindsley's *activation* theory, and Papez's *limbic* theory of emotion (Cannon, 1931: 281–95; Lindsley, 1951:504–9; Papez, 1937:725–43).

Lindsley's non-specific activation theory has been well substantiated with respect to correlation of the quantitative aspects of emotional excitation with levels of non-specific activation. Table VIII adapted from Lindsley (1960:1554) summarizes these findings.

Lindsley's non-specific activation theory directly accounts for the excitement-quietude emotional aspects of perception and behavior. The theory might also be interpreted to mean that pleasure is a function of low to moderate levels of arousal while unpleasure is a function of excessively augmented levels. However, since raucous hilarity as well as drowsy comfort can be extremely pleasurable, pleasure clearly is not a simple equivalent of low levels of arousal activation. Similarly, since states of lethargic depression as well as of excited panic can be extremely unpleasurable, unpleasure clearly is not a simple equivalent of elevated arousal activation. Pleasure and unpleasure apparently are at least partially independent of states of general arousal.

The theory that pleasure and unpleasure are functions of u-h-r discharge via *unique* patterns of phasic non-specific activation accounts for the partial *independence* of pleasure and unpleasure from states of excitability and arousal. Its tenet that pleasure, unpleasure, and arousal are all derivatives of non-specific activation accounts for their *interdependence*.

Summary

According to the hypotheses presented in this chapter, the reverberatory u-h-r system circuits discharge not only via (1) tonic and phasic ascending non-specific *arousal* activation of perceptual consciousness and wakeful behavior, but also (2) unique patterns of phasic ascending non-specific *pleasure and unpleasure* activation of perceptual consciousness and wakeful behavior.

---

[*] Erogenous sensation and pleasure would be differentiable on the same basis of an extrinsic-sensory versus an intrinsic-reverberatory input.

Chapter IV

Upper Limbic-Hypothalamic-Reticular
Contributions to
Extrapyramidal Rhythmic Movements

Chapters IV, V, and VI deal respectively with the discharge of the u-h-r circuits via extrapyramidal rhythmic movements, generalized states of muscular tonus, and visceral and endocrine reactions. In Chapters VII and VIII these considerations will lead to the development of a theory of emotion as a function of u-h-r circuit discharge via six different avenues of activation.

An understanding of u-h-r contributions to extrapyramidal postures and rhythmic movements requires some reference to the functions of the extrapyramidal system. Figure IV-1 depicts prominent components of the extrapyramidal system. Figures IV-2, IV-6, IV-7, and IV-8 direct attention to its spinal and cranial distribution via respectively the descending reticulospinal tracts and the cranial nerves.

The extrapyramidal system is a "non-specific" motor system in that it is involved with states of generalized muscular tonus or with diffuse repetitive motor patterns such as locomotion or swinging of the arms, in which there is a paucity of demarcated change from one block of time to another (House and Pansky, 1967:366). Its functions contrast with those of the pyramidal motor system, which is characterized by specificity with respect to both its highly demarcated topographic organization within areas 4 and 6 of the cortex (Fig. IV-3) and its involvement with extremely demarcated precise and localized movements of individual muscles.

The Lower Extrapyramidal System

The lower extrapyramidal system, located within the midbrain, pons, and medulla, consists primarily of the following groups of nuclei:

Lower Extrapyramidal Nuclei Whose Discharge Primarily Affects the Musculature of the Head

The motor nuclei of the cranial nerves (Figs. IV-6 and IV-8) serve as lower extrapyramidal stations for the distribution of impulses to the mus-

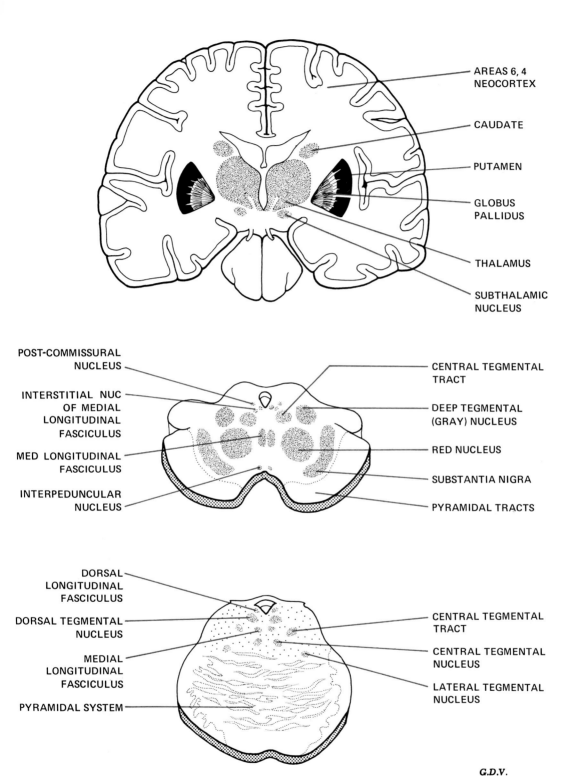

AREAS 6, 4
NEOCORTEX

CAUDATE

PUTAMEN

GLOBUS
PALLIDUS

THALAMUS

SUBTHALAMIC
NUCLEUS

POST-COMMISSURAL
NUCLEUS

INTERSTITIAL NUC
OF MEDIAL
LONGITUDINAL
FASCICULUS

MED LONGITUDINAL
FASCICULUS

INTERPEDUNCULAR
NUCLEUS

CENTRAL TEGMENTAL
TRACT

DEEP TEGMENTAL
(GRAY) NUCLEUS

RED NUCLEUS

SUBSTANTIA NIGRA

PYRAMIDAL TRACTS

DORSAL
LONGITUDINAL
FASCICULUS

DORSAL TEGMENTAL
NUCLEUS

MEDIAL
LONGITUDINAL
FASCICULUS

PYRAMIDAL SYSTEM

CENTRAL TEGMENTAL
TRACT

CENTRAL TEGMENTAL
NUCLEUS

LATERAL TEGMENTAL
NUCLEUS

G.D.V.

Figure IV-1. Prominent components of the extrapyramidal motor system.

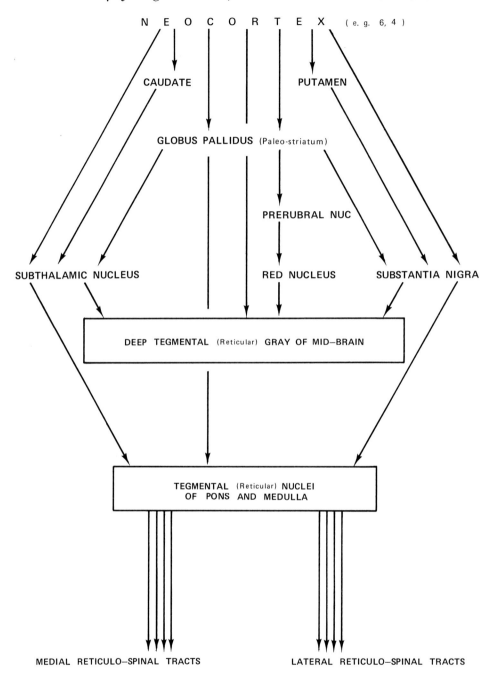

Figure IV-2. Prominent components of the extrapyramidal motor system which discharge via the reticulo-spinal tracts to supply the musculature of the limbs and body proper.

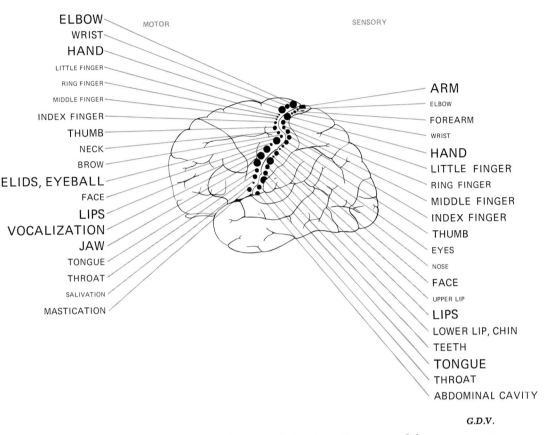

ELBOW
WRIST
HAND
LITTLE FINGER
RING FINGER
MIDDLE FINGER
INDEX FINGER
THUMB
NECK
BROW
ELIDS, EYEBALL
FACE
LIPS
VOCALIZATION
JAW
TONGUE
THROAT
SALIVATION
MASTICATION

MOTOR   SENSORY

ARM
ELBOW
FOREARM
WRIST
HAND
LITTLE FINGER
RING FINGER
MIDDLE FINGER
INDEX FINGER
THUMB
EYES
NOSE
FACE
UPPER LIP
LIPS
LOWER LIP, CHIN
TEETH
TONGUE
THROAT
ABDOMINAL CAVITY

G.D.V.

Figure IV-3. The topographical localization of the "specific" pyramidal motor system and of the specific somaesthetic-proprioceptive sensory systems within the cerebral cortex.

culature of the face and neck, including the musculature of the eyes, jaw, tongue, and larynx, and thereby mediate extrapyramidal control of eye movements, mastication, and phonation (Crosby, 1962:255, Fig. 192; House and Pansky, 1967:222).

Lower Extrapyramidal Nuclei Whose Discharge Primarily Affects Extension, Flexion, and Rotation of the Limbs and Body Proper as well as Respiration

The reticular, tegmental, motor nuclei are the lower extrapyramidal stations for the distribution of impulses to the musculature of the limbs and body proper. They serve as a funnel for the transmission of impulses from upper and middle extrapyramidal areas into the descending reticulo-spinal tracts which innervate the musculature at spinal levels. (see Figs. IV-2, IV-6, and IV-7).

Figure IV-4 schematically illustrates the relation of these nuclei to extension and flexion (see House and Pansky, 1967:378–83; Ruch, 1965:216–17; and Eldred and Fujimori, 1958:275–82).

The diagram draws attention to the following information:

1. The lower extrapyramidal system includes on the left and right the following reticulo-motor areas or "nuclei":

    a. extensor facilitatory nuclei
    b. flexor facilitatory nuclei
    c. extensor inhibitory nuclei
    d. flexor inhibitory nuclei

2. Pathways from these nuclei converge upon the descending reticulo-spinal tracts.

3. The reticulo-spinal tracts in turn distribute collaterals to the extensor and flexor stretch reflex arcs at all spinal levels (see French, 1960:1291–3). Figure IV-4 illustrates ipsilateral reticulo-spinal connections of the extensor facilitatory nuclei with extensor reflex arcs and of the flexor facilitatory nuclei with flexor reflex arcs. These connections provide a possible route by which stimulation of the extensor facilitatory nuclei results in the discharge of impulses to all ipsilateral extensors, and stimulation of the flexor facilitatory nuclei results in the discharge of impulses to all ipsilateral flexors.

4. The extensor and flexor inhibitory nuclei discharge via an equivalent route (ibid:1291–2).

5. In addition, the diagram peripherally refers to lower extrapyramidal rotator and vital respiratory nuclei. These, like the extensor and flexor nuclei, connect with the descending reticulo-spinal tracts. Lower extrapyramidal facilitation or inhibition of rotation or respiration is made possible by connections of these tracts with spinal reflex arcs of the rotator and of the respiratory musculature (see review by Jung and Hassler, 1960:896, Fig. 11; and by French, 1960:1295; House and Pansky, 1967:211–12; Oberholzer, 1960:1112).

Middle Extrapyramidal System

Neuroanatomical Considerations

Numerous middle extrapyramidal nuclei serve prominent roles in the organization of rhythmic behavior. Among these are the red nucleus, substantia nigra, and subthalamic nucleus, each connecting with different groups of lower extrapyramidal reticulo-motor nuclei (Figs. IV-2, IV-6, and IV-7), and the interpeduncular, interstitial, and post-commissural nuclei each connecting with groups of motor nuclei of the cranial nerves

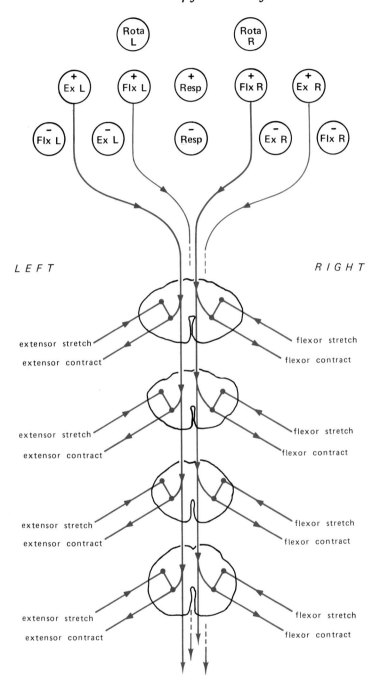

EAG

Figure IV-4. Extension and flexion in relation to the reticular motor nuclei.

(Figs. IV-6 and IV-8). As previously noted, impulses from the middle extrapyramidal nuclei are transmitted to the lower extrapyramidal motor nuclei and thence, via the cranial nerves and the reticulo-spinal tracts, to the musculature of the head, limbs, and body proper.

Functional Properties of the Middle Extrapyramidal System

Studies of brain pathology reveal that the functions of the middle extrapyramidal nuclei involve the discharge of diffuse repetitive motor rhythmic reactions. For example, rhythmic tremors as found in parkinsonism are associated with lesions of the substantia nigra, while swinging of the arms in rolling wave-like twisting patterns (hemiballism) is associated with disturbances of the subthalamic nuclei (House and Pansky, 1967:386–8). The extrapyramidal system sets up approximate positions of the body parts through the adjustment of large muscle groups and thereby mediates semiautomatic movements such as swinging the arms and locomotion (ibid: 366–7).

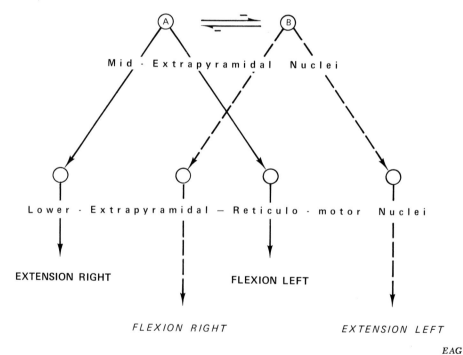

EAG

Figure IV-5. Intrinsic, mid-extrapyramidal regulation of rythmic movement.

Figure IV-5 presents a schema which would account for the organization of rhythmic movements on the basis of connections between middle and lower extrapyramidal motor nuclei (see de Long, 1971:10–30). The process is comparable to a pianist's rendition of a musical phrase as he repeats certain selected notes from the total piano keyboard. The different lower extrapyramidal reticular motor nuclei whose discharge affects the total body musculature are the equivalent of the musical keyboard. A group of these lower extrapyramidal nuclei may be repetitively "played upon" via alternating innervation of different connections from the middle extrapyramidal nuclei. This formulation of extrapyramidal functioning reflects Hess' conclusions (see Jung and Hassler, 1960:896) that descending mesencephalic, mid-extrapyramidal processes may serve as a "selecting organ," selectively inhibiting or facilitating specific reactions associated with lower extrapyramidal reticulo-motor nuclei. In accord with such a formulation, intrinsic contributions to patterned movement characteristic of locomotion would be understandable in terms of the schema in Figure IV-5.

The schema demonstrates a reciprocally antithetical interaction between A and B so that discharge of A via

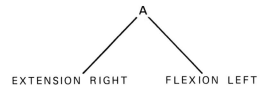

alternates with the discharge of B via

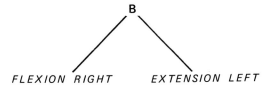

Such "built-in" intrinsic middle extrapyramidal regulation of locomotion may substitute for extrinsic stimulus effects. The spinal reflex components of locomotion which may be set in motion by extrinsic stimulus patterns may be intrinsically activated if the central nervous system at the level of the red nucleus has been left intact (see Eldred, 1960:1080, 1084).

The conceptualization suggested by Figure IV-5 applies also to middle extrapyramidal rhythmical innervation of the lower extrapyramidal inspiratory and expiratory motor nuclei (see Oberholzer, 1960:1118 and Fig. 4). Presumably mid-extrapyramidal eye, head, and jaw movements are organized on a similar basis.

Upper Extrapyramidal System

The specific distribution of connections between upper and middle extrapyramidal nuclei (Figs. IV-2, IV-6, IV-7, and IV-8) provides a route by which impulses descending from upper extrapyramidal areas may selectively facilitate and inhibit a number of middle extrapyramidal patterns of rhythmic movement (French, 1960:1295–6). These upper extrapyramidal inhibitory and facilitatory processes offer a source for stop and go effects upon a number of different middle extrapyramidal patterns of rhythmic movement. Jung and Hassler (1960:874) summarize findings from the experimental literature which indicate that destruction of the caudate nucleus and putamen actually does result in the loss of stop and go control of extrapyramidal rhythmic behavior: such lesions, for example, eventuate in an irresistible drive of animal subjects to run straight forward regardless of obstacles. These effects upon rhythmic movement apparently also pertain to responses released at cranial levels: lesions of the basal ganglia have been found to cause severe disturbances in the regulation of feeding mechanisms, visual coordination, and speech (ibid:914).

The anatomical structure of the basal ganglia and premotor cortex furthermore offers a source for upper extrapyramidal spatial patterning of rhythmic movements. Extrapyramidal representation within the basal ganglia and premotor cortex is characterized by somatotopic localization. Forman and Ward (1957:230) note that within the caudate nucleus, foci affecting turning of the head, neck, trunk, or legs are respectively situated adjacent to one another. This organization would make possible a spatial as well as temporal coordination of middle extrapyramidal rhythms affecting different parts of the body.

U-H-R Circuit Discharge via Extrapyramidal Rhythmic Movement: Neuroanatomical Evidence

Prominent anatomical paths connecting the u-h-r system circuits with specific groups of upper, middle, and lower extrapyramidal nuclei are shown in Figures IV-6, IV-7, and IV-8.

These findings draw attention to the multiplicity of u-h-r connections with the extrapyramidal motor system at all levels. One would therefore predict that discharge of the u-h-r circuits must activate a variety of extrapyramidal postures and repetitive rhythmic movements as well as more complex extrapyramidal patterns of behavior. These postures and movements would be expected to involve the musculature of both the body proper (locomotion, turning, rolling, breathing) and of the cranium (mastication, swallowing, phonation, posturing and movements of the eyes and head).

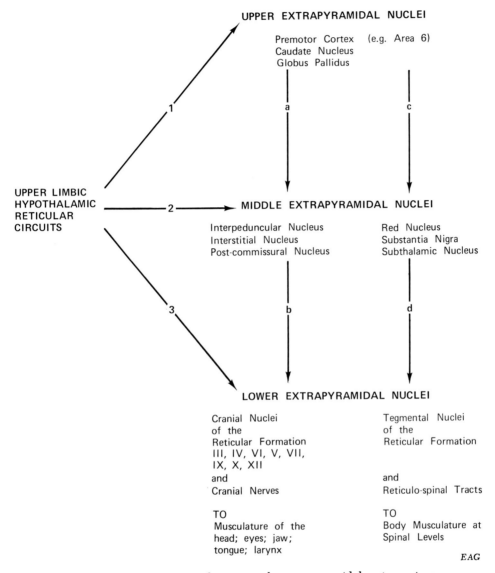

Figure IV-6. U-H-R contributions to the extrapyramidal motor system.

Figure IV-6 References: Letters and numbers refer to tracts listed in Figure IV-6.

    a. Jung and Hassler, 1960:891, Fig. 8; Kappers, 1936:1081.

    b. Crosby, Humphrey and Lauer, 1962:254–5; House and Pansky, 1967:222; Jung and Hassler, 1960:891, Fig. 8; Kappers, 1936:1079.

    c, d. see Fig. IV-3; House and Pansky, 1967:367–82.

  1. Jung and Hassler, 1960:920; House and Pansky, 1967:367 (footnote 7), 368.

  2. Kappers, 1936:1102, 1101–3, 1083; House and Pansky, 1967:221–2.

  3. Ingram, 1960:964; House and Pansky, 1967:409–10; Kappers, 1936:1182; Crosby, 1962:319.

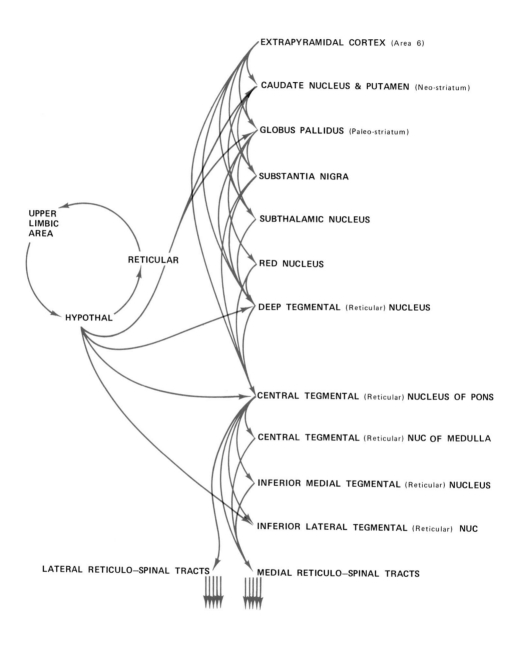

EAG

Figure IV-7. U-H-R contributions (red) to the extrapyramidal motor system (green): spinal distribution via the reticulo-spinal tracts.

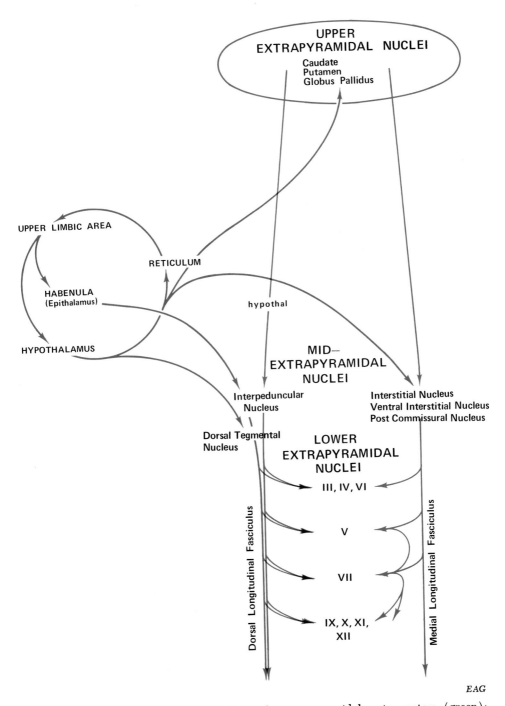

Figure IV-8. U-H-R contributions (red) to the extrapyramidal motor system (green): cranial distribution via the cranial nerves.

TABLE IX
U-H-R SYSTEM DISCHARGE VIA EXTRAPYRAMIDAL RHYTHMIC MOVEMENTS

Area Studied	Reference	Experimental Technique	Extrapyramidal Rhythmic Movements and Postures Activated
1. HYPOTHALAMUS			
Anterior sectors	Delgado, 1967:66	Electrode stimulation in monkeys	Walking, climbing, flapping of ears, vocalization
Posterior sectors	Ibid:66	Electrode stimulation in monkeys	Turning, rubbing
2. UPPER LIMBIC AREA			
Septal nuclei	Eliasson with reference to Hess and Magnus, 1960:1165	Electrode stimulation	Chewing
Hippocampus	Delgado, 1967:66	Electrical stimulation in monkeys	Running
Amygdala	See Gloor, 1960:1404	Electrode stimulation in freely moving animals	Circling, rolling; flexion and extension of limbs; turning of head and eyes
	See Gloor, ibid:1404	Electrode stimulation in animals	Change in rhythm, amplitude, and position of thorax during respiration; sneezing, sniffing, coughing
	MacLean and Delgado, 1953:91	Electrode stimulation among cats	Searching and arrest of head and eyes; swallowing, licking, chewing, biting, grunting, hissing
	Delgado, 1967:66	Electrode stimulation of monkeys	Crouching, abnormal postures
Pyriform cortex	See Kaada, 1960:1351	Electrode stimulation in cats	Acceleration of respiration
	See Kaada, ibid:1357	Electrode stimulation in monkeys, cats and dogs	Chewing
Cingulate cortex	See Kaada, ibid:1357	Electrode stimulation among monkeys	Vocalization
Orbito-frontal cortex	See Kaada, ibid:1361	Electrode stimulation	Arrest and searching of head and eyes
	Langworthy and Richter, 1939:158—61	Bilateral removal	Prolonged locomotion

U-H-R Circuit Discharge
via Extrapyramidal Rhythmic Movement:
Neurophysiological Evidence

The typical neurophysiological findings presented in Table IX substantiate conclusions drawn from anatomical studies that the hypothalamic and upper limbic components of the u-h-r circuits discharge via extrapyramidal rhythmic movements and postures at spinal and cranial levels.

Thus, both neuroanatomical and neurophysiological studies indicate the u-h-r system circuits connect with and discharge via the extrapyramidal motor system, a basis for the activation of a variety of postures and rhythmic movements.

In summary, the u-h-r system circuits discharge via contributions to (1) tonic and phasic ascending non-specific arousal activation of perceptual consciousness and wakeful behavior, (2) patterned phasic ascending non-specific pleasure and unpleasure activation of perceptual consciousness and behavior, and (3) extrapyramidal postures and rhythmic movements.

Chapter V

Upper Limbic-Hypothalamic-Reticular Contributions to Descending Tonic Non-Specific Activation

An understanding of u-h-r contributions to descending non-specific activation requires some reference to the neuroanatomical and physiological characteristics of descending non-specific activation.

The Reticular Formation in Relation to Descending Tonic Non-specific Activation

The Reticular Formation as an Internuncial System

Reference has been made to reticular sensory functions in relation to non-specific fusion of sensory impulses from all sections of the body and from all modalities (see French, 1960:1284). On the other hand, the reticular formation has been described as primarily "a motor-coordinating center, the lower part for respiration, the higher parts for eye movements and body posture" (Jung and Hassler, 1960:913). Confusion may arise as to how primary functions of the reticular formation can be both sensory and motor. French (ibid:1282) resolves this confusion as he points to experimental findings indicating that embryologically the reticular system is basically neither motor nor sensory, but is an internuncial, interconnecting system. House and Pansky (1967:378) make reference to this concept: "The reticular formation is spread throughout the brainstem between the tracts and nuclei thereof, making up the bulk of tissue in the central portions of the tegmentum of the medulla, pons, and mid-brain. Originally it consisted mainly of the axons of association neurons interconnecting sensory and motor nuclei. Later in phylogenesis . . . nuclear groups developed within the fibrous reticulum." Among these groups are sensory nuclei as well as the motor nuclei of the extrapyramidal system.

Reticulo-Motor Nuclei Enmeshed Within the Internuncial Reticular Formation

Enmeshed within the internuncial reticular formation are (1) the extrapyramidal extensor, flexor, rotator, and respiratory nuclei mediating discharge of behavior at spinal levels (see Figs. IV–4 and V–1 and Eldred and Fujimori, 1958:278–82; Jung and Hassler, 1960:895, Fig. 11; Ruch, 1965: 217), and (2) the motor nuclei of the cranial nerves mediating extrapyramidal discharge of behavior at cranial levels. Scheibel and Scheibel (1958: 41) note: "In addition to the innumerable synaptic connections with reticular elements at other levels, most reticular axons have been shown by both histologic and physiologic methods to project to nuclei of the cranial nerves. Such collaterals may come off at any point along the axon . . . The reticulo-nuclear collaterals may arborize widely in three dimensions within the cranial nucleus often producing almost as exuberant a plexus as a sensory presynaptic terminal. We have now seen collaterals of reticular axons enter all cranial nerve nuclei of the medulla, pons, and mesencephalon . . . So far as we can see, the terminating reticular collaterals effect synaptic contact with both dendrites and somata of the cranial nuclei."

The diagram in Figure V–1 schematically depicts (1) the internuncial reticulum within which the cranial and spinal divisions of the lower extrapyramidal nuclei are enmeshed, (2) the input into the reticulum, sources for its activation or "charge," and (3) the output or discharge of the reticulum via these extrapyramidal nuclei, the cranial nerves,[*] and the descending reticulo-spinal tracts.

Descending Non-specific Activation, a Derivative of Non-specific Internuncial Activation of the Reticular Motor Nuclei

Fig. V–1 demonstrates (1) the internuncial reticulum is charged via the extrinsic sensory system and via the intrinsic u-h-r system circuits; (2) this non-specific state of activation of the reticulum is then distributed diffusely not only upwards to the cerebral cortex but also directly to the numerous reticular motor nuclei. These nuclei become activated en masse: there occurs equal internuncial activation of the reticular nuclei for flexion, extension, and turning, on the right and on the left, of spinal and cranial portions of the body. The maintenance of such diffuse tonically non-specific activation in turn results in a state of immobilization. For, if flexion, extension, and rotation to the left and to the right at spinal and cranial levels are all equally activated, then a rigid, equally balanced state of activation of all musculature and of all muscular reflexes occurs. The consequent simultaneous contraction of opposing muscle groups eventuates in joints becoming fixed and pillar-like (see Ruch, 1965:216–219). The picture resulting from such diffuse activation of the reticular motor nuclei, then, would be expected to be that of decerebrate rigidity. And in actuality, uninhibited exposure of reticulo-motor discharge patterns following brainstem transection does eventuate in decerebrate rigidity.

[*] Not depicted in Figure V–1.

Furthermore, enmeshed within the reticular formation are the inhibitory as well as facilitatory flexor and extensor nuclei (Eldred and Fujimori, 1958: 275–82). Tonic non-specific internuncial activation of the total assembly of reticular motor nuclei therefore is distributed not only to (1) all facilitatory extensor and flexor reticular nuclei, a source for interlocked, immobile, pillar-like rigidity, but also to (2) all inhibitory extensor and flexor reticular nuclei, a source for reduced forcefulness of extensor and flexor muscular contraction. A state of complete muscular rigidity thereby becomes attenuated and converted into balanced muscular relaxation and plasticity.

Internuncial activation of the reticular nuclei thus eventuates in descending non-specific activation: (1) *non-specific* in the sense that (a) impulses from both extrinsic and intrinsic sources become fused within the diffuse reticulum and (b) all reticular motor nuclei are non-specifically activated at once; (2) *descending* in the sense that activated impulses from these lower extrapyramidal reticular nuclei are transmitted to the total body musculature via the cranial motor nerves and descending reticulo-spinal tracts.

U-H-R Contributions to
Tonic Descending Non-specific Activation

If activation of the internuncial reticular formation results in descending non-specific activation of the total body musculature, then u-h-r discharge via the reticular formation should affect the level of descending non-specific activation and, therefore, should influence the magnitude of generalized muscular tonicity and tension. Neurophysiological findings confirm this conclusion:

Orbital-Insular-Temporal Cortices: Kaada (1960:1352) reports that electrical stimulation within these upper limbic areas results in a generalized inhibition of reflexes and widespread muscular relaxation. Eyelids close, arms and legs become limp.

Amygdala: Gloor (1960:1404) refers to a number of experimental studies indicating that electrode stimulation of the amygdala results in a generalized increase in muscle tone as well as the arrest of spontaneous movements. Spinal reflexes are facilitated or inhibited depending upon what areas of the amygdala are stimulated.

Hypothalamus: Hess (see Jung and Hassler, 1960:912) has shown that coagulation of the posterior hypothalamus bordering the reticular formation eventuates in a syndrome characterized by a loss of muscle tone.

Thus both anatomical and physiological findings indicate that the upper limbic, hypothalamic, and reticular components of the u-h-r system circuits discharge via descending (+ / −) activation of muscular tonus.

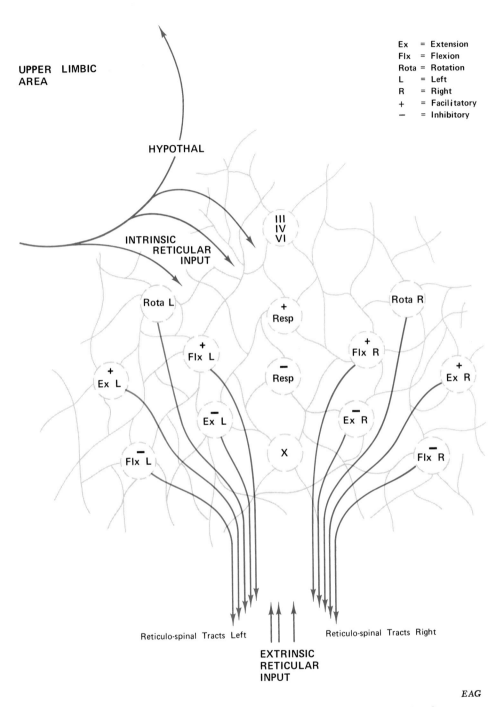

Figure V-1. Lower extrapyramidal motor nuclei enmeshed within the brainstem reticulum. (See Fig. IV-4)

In summary, the u-h-r system circuits discharge via contributions to (1) tonic and phasic ascending non-specific arousal activation of perceptual consciousness and wakeful behavior, (2) patterned phasic ascending non-specific pleasure and unpleasure activation of perceptual consciousness and behavior, (3) extrapyramidal postures and rhythmic movements, and (4) tonic descending non-specific activation of general muscular tone and tension.

Chapter VI

Upper Limbic-Hypothalamic-Reticular System Circuit Contributions to Autonomic-Visceral and Pituitary-Endocrine Discharge

U-H-R DISCHARGE VIA AUTONOMIC NERVOUS SYSTEM

Neurological studies involving respectively the (1) reticular formation, (2) hypothalamus, and (3) upper limbic areas indicate that each of these components of the u-h-r circuit systems is connected with the autonomic visceral nervous system.

The Reticular Formation: Visceral Connections

Embedded within the internuncial network of the reticular tegmentum are not only the somatic nuclei of the lower extrapyramidal motor system, but also autonomic nuclei of the sympathetic and parasympathetic nervous systems. Most prominent among these are the following:

1. The facilitatory and inhibitory vasomotor nuclei which mediate reflexes pertaining to vasculature constriction (see Ingram, 1960:958).

2. Facilitatory and inhibitory inspiratory nuclei* (ibid:959).

3. Facilitatory and inhibitory sudomotor nuclei which mediate reflexes pertaining to sweat gland secretion (ibid:961).

4. The dorsal tegmental nucleus whose discharge via the descending dorsal longitudinal fasciculus is distributed to the total thoraco-lumbar chain of sympathetic ganglia (see ibid:961; Kappers, 1936:1083–5).

5. The dorsal nucleus of the vagus whose discharge via the parasympathetic fibres of the vagus is distributed to the principal viscera within the thoracic and abdominal cavities (see Scheibel and Scheibel, 1958:42; House and Pansky, 1967:335).

6. The salivatory nuclei whose discharge innervates secretion of the salivary glands (Crosby, 1962:157 Fig. 132).

Tonic non-specific internuncial activation of the total assembly of reticular sympathetic and parasympathetic motor nuclei therefore should result

*These nuclei belong to both the extrapyramidal-somatic and the autonomic-visceral systems.

in the diffuse reinforcement of all facilitatory and inhibitory visceral reflexes. In this way the processes of descending reticular non-specific visceral activation parallel those of descending reticular non-specific somatic activation (Ingram, 1960:961). The diagram in Figure VI–1 schematically illustrates activation of the visceral systems via the reticular formation.

The Hypothalamic and Upper Limbic Areas: Autonomic Visceral Connections

The hypothalamus and upper limbic areas are connected with the reticular visceral motor nuclei via numerous tracts including the medial forebrain bundle and the periventricular system (see Ingram, 1960:964–5; Kappers, 1936:1101–3, 1083–4, 1182).

These neuroanatomical findings lead to the expectation that hypothalamic and upper limbic discharge should contribute to reticular specific activation of visceral reactions. Neurophysiological studies such as those carried out by Hess (1954) confirm this hypothesis. Hess found that electrode stimulation of the posterior hypothalamus elicits an array of sympathetic visceral reactions: pupillary dilitation, rise in blood pressure, increase in pulse rate, and a rise in the respiratory rate. Electrode stimulation of the more anterior portions of the hypothalamus elicits the discharge of parasympathetic visceral reactions: pupillary contraction, a drop in arterial blood pressure, a decrease in the respiratory rate, salivation, micturation, and defecation.

With respect to functions of the upper limbic areas, electrode stimulation of the orbital, temporal, cingulate, and hippocampal cortices and the associated amygdaloid and septal areas results in facilitatory and inhibitory effects upon all phases of autonomic balance: gastrointestinal reactions, arterial pressure, peripheral vasomotor tone, respiration, pupillary reactions, and sweating (see French, 1960:1299–1300).

In summary, both neuroanatomical and neurophysiological findings pertaining to the upper limbic areas as well as to the hypothalamus and reticular formation lead to the conclusion that the u-h-r system circuits, at all levels, discharge via descending visceral activation.

DISCHARGE OF THE U-H-R SYSTEM CIRCUITS VIA DESCENDING PITUITARY ACTIVATION

Neuroanatomical Considerations

Hypothalamic discharge has been shown to affect pituitary gland secretion (Harris, 1960:1007–34). A rich portal vascular system, likened to that of the liver, has been described as interconnecting the hypothalamus and pituitary gland, and, according to mounting but still incomplete evidence, it is via hypothalamic neurosecretion into this portal system that CNS con-

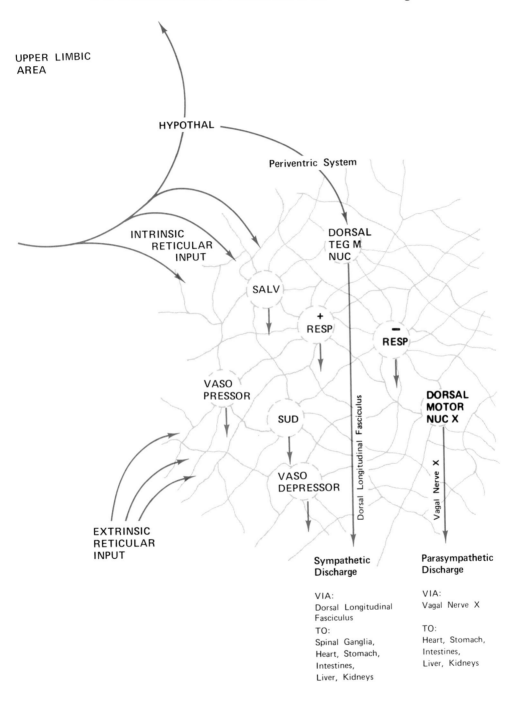

Figure VI-1. Autonomic nuclei enmeshed within the brainstem reticulum.

trol of anterior pituitary functions is mediated (ibid:1010–11). Harris' original findings directed attention to the accessibility of the hypothalamic pituitary portal system for neurosecretory transmission. Arterial twigs from the internal carotid and posterior communicating arteries form a rich vascular plexus over the surface of the median eminence of the hypothalamus. Myriads of capillary loops from this plexus become entwined with the neurosecretory axons of the hypothalamus and therefore are in a position to absorb chemical substances secreted by these axons. The capillary loops then coalesce into larger trunks which pass down the hypophysial stalk and drain into the sinusoids of the anterior lobe of the pituitary gland. Figure VI–2 depicts the transmission of neurosecretions from hypothalamus to anterior pituitary via this localized capillary system.

Neurophysiological Considerations

On the basis of the connections between hypothalamus and pituitary, hypothalamic discharge should exert an influence upon reactions of the pituitary gland regulating the processes of the adrenal cortex, testes, ovaries, and thyroid. Neurophysiological studies substantiate this conclusion:

Hypothalamic Discharge via the Pituitary Gland: Activation of the Adrenocorticotrophic Hormone

Electrical stimulation of the hypothalamus results in pituitary discharge of ACTH, the adrenocorticotrophic hormone, into the bloodstream so as to activate the steroid hormones of the adrenal cortex (see Harris, 1960:1025). Hans Selye's studies of "the stress syndrome" contribute to a realization of the vast significance of this process whereby hypothalamic discharge affects the production of the adrenal cortical hormones (see Magda Arnold, 1960: 237). His studies reveal that the release of ACTH from the anterior pituitary into the bloodstream stimulates the secretion of two groups of hormones from the cortex of the adrenal glands. One group which includes cortisone and cortisol *counteracts inflammation;* the other group which includes desoxycorticosterone and aldosterone *promotes inflammation.* Both the pro-inflammatory and anti-inflammatory processes normally serve the body's defense against disease. Inflammation walls off invading organisms or foreign substances while reduced inflammation is required once the pathological organisms or substances have been controlled. However, both the pro-inflammatory and the anti-inflammatory adrenal cortical hormones can themselves produce disease. When invading substances are harmless, inflammation interferes with health as in hayfever, infantile eczema, asthma, bursitis, and arthritis. On the other hand, when infection is active, reduction of inflammatory reactions leave the patient vulnerable to the spread of disease which in extreme cases may cause death (ibid:237–42).

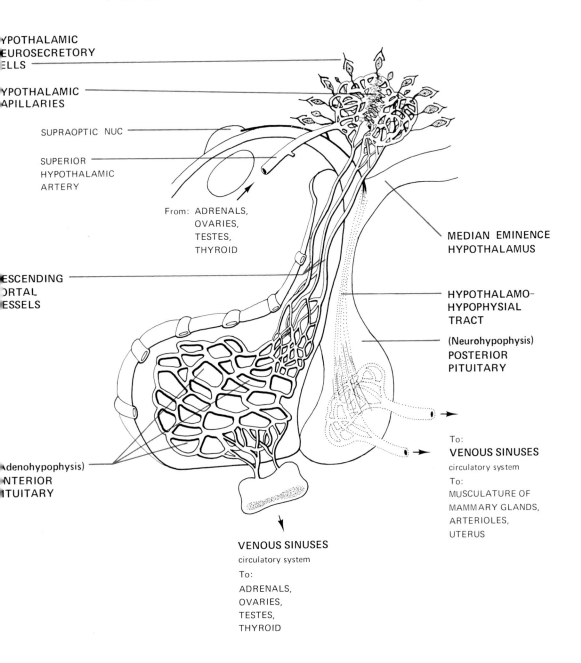

Figure VI-2. The hypothalamic-hypophysial portal system.

The discharge of the hypothalamic component of the u-h-r system circuits, therefore, may vitally affect the psychosomatic adjustment of the organism by overactivating or inhibiting ACTH and thereby precipitating inflammatory disturbances or reducing the subject's resistance to infection.

Hypothalamic Discharge via the Pituitary Gland: Activation of the Gonadotrophic, Lactogenic and Thyrotrophic Hormones

(1) Harris (1960:1011) showed as early as 1937 that electrical stimulation of the hypothalamus excites gonadotrophic hormones. These findings have continued to be confirmed by researchers such as McCann (Watanabe and McCann, 1968:664–73; Crighton, Schneider, and McCann, 1970:328–9) who have begun to localize hypothalamic sites which release neurosecretions regulating the pituitary gonadotrophic hormones. (2) Evidence has been accumulating which indicates that a neurosecretion from the hypothalamus controls (inhibits) prolactin, the lactogenic hormone of the anterior pituitary which activates the mammary secretion of milk. (Meites, 1966:688–90). (3) Harris' (see 1960:1025) experimental studies have revealed that electrical stimulation of certain areas of the hypothalamus results in increased thyroid activity. Bowers (1970:1143–53) and Burgus (1970: 321–25) have recently been able to identify as a tripeptide the hypothalamic neurosecretion which activates the pituitary thyrotrophic hormones.

Upper Limbic Discharge via the Pituitary Gland

On the basis of connections of the upper limbic areas with the hypothalamus, and the hypothalamus with the pituitary, the reactions of the pituitary gland should also be able to be influenced by impulses descending from the upper limbic areas. Table X refers to a sample of experimental studies which confirm this conclusion.

These findings lead to the conclusion that the hypothalamic and upper limbic components of the u-h-r system circuits discharge via the pituitary portal system and activate the anterior pituitary trophic hormones.* In this way, u-h-r system discharge affects reproductive processes as well as the capacity of the organism to react to stress and disease.

In summary, available evidence indicates that the u-h-r system circuits may discharge via (1) tonic and phasic ascending non-specific arousal activation of perceptual consciousness and wakeful behavior, (2) patterned phasic ascending non-specific pleasure and unpleasure activation of perceptual consciousness and behavior, (3) extrapyramidal postures and rhythmic movements, (4) tonic descending non-specific activation of general muscular tone and tension, (5) descending activation of sym-

---

* Discharge of the u-h-r circuits via the posterior pituitary is considered in Chapter IX.

TABLE X
U-H-R SYSTEM DISCHARGE VIA PITUITARY GLAND ACTIVATION

Area	Reference	Experimental Procedure	Pituitary Effects
Amygdala	Mangili, 1966:316	Bilateral lesions	Reduction of pituitary effects upon the adrenal cortex
	Bunn, 1957:369—71	Electrode stimulation	Gonadotrophic induction of ovulation
	Elwers, 1961:281—84	Interruption of the stria terminalis	Precocious ovarian development
Hippocampus	See Shadé, 1970:5—6	Electrode stimulation	Inhibition of ACTH release
	See Shadé, 1970:6	Bilateral lesions	Elevation of plasma level of corticoids
	Kawakami, 1967:99—100	Electrode stimulation	Gonadotrophic induction of ovulation in estrogen-primed rabbits
		Electrode stimulation	Enhanced formation of progesterone
Septal nuclei	Heath, 1954:306	Electrode stimulation	Elevated adrenal cortical activity (as evidenced by marked decrease in blood lymphocytes)

pathetic and parasympathetic visceral reactions, and (6) descending pituitary activation.

Figure VI–3 refers schematically to these avenues of discharge.

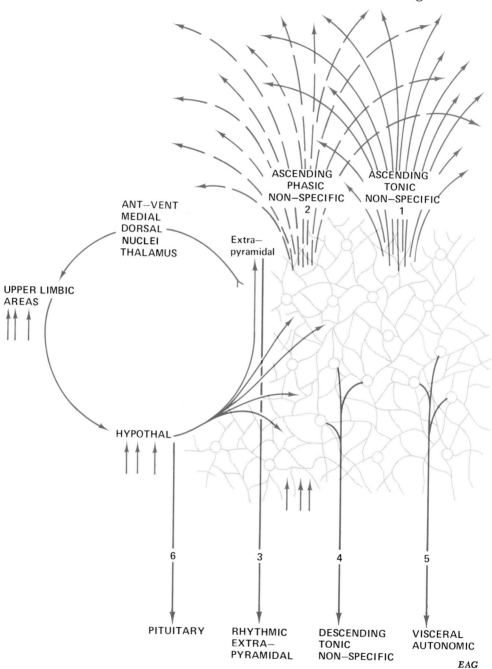

Figure VI-3. The discharge of the u-h-r systems via six avenues of activation.

Chapter VII

The Upper Limbic-Hypothalamic-Reticular Somatic Arousal System, Visceral Arousal System, and the Pleasure-Unpleasure System

The u-h-r systems whose *physiological* properties have been reviewed in the preceding chapters may be classified in terms of their *psychological* effects upon behavior:

1. A Somatic Arousal System which discharges via ascending and descending non-specific activation and via the innervation of extrapyramidal rhythmic movements of the skeletal musculature.

2. A Pleasure-Unpleasure System which presumably discharges via patterns of ascending phasic non-specific activation.

3. A Visceral Arousal System which discharges via descending sympathetic and parasympathetic autonomic reactions as well as via pituitary activation.

The Somatic Arousal System

The Somatic Arousal System consists of facilitatory and inhibitory components. Reference has already been made to upper limbic, hypothalamic, and reticular foci whose stimulation elicits facilitatory effects upon non-specific arousal of consciousness and wakeful behavior. This facilitatory system has been referred to by a number of different names: the Wakefulness (Nauta, 1946:285), the Dynamogenic (Hess, 1954:117), and the Vigilance Systems (Hernandez-Peon, 1964:210).

Conversely, stimulation of other upper limbic, hypothalamic, and reticular foci inhibits non-specific arousal activation of consciousness and wakeful behavior. When these inhibitory effects are maximal, they eventuate in a state of sleep (e.g., Nauta, 1946:285, Hernandez-Peon and Chavez-Ibarra, 1963:197–8). This inhibitory system has been referred to as the Hypnogenic System (Hess, 1954:117), and as the Sleep System or Center (see Hernandez-Peon, 1964:211, Fig. 15; Nauta, 1946:285). The term "Tranquilizing

71

System" also is appropriate since it conveys the concept of a reduction in non-specific arousal activation which does not necessarily eventuate in a state of sleep.

The Pleasure and Unpleasure System

The properties of the non-specific Pleasure and Unpleasure System have been considered in Chapters I through III. This system may also be referred to as the Reward and Punishment System since pleasure and reward, like unpleasure and punishment, are conjoint functions (see Chapter XI).

The Visceral Arousal System

Cannon (1939) drew attention to the emergency and vegetative functions of the sympathetic and parasympathetic visceral autonomic nervous systems. Hess (1954) has used the rather elaborate terms "Ergotrophic" and "Trophotrophic" to refer to the central u-h-r organization of these sympathetic-emergency and parasympathetic-vegetative functions.

The U-H-R Systems:
General Properties

Since the Somatic and Visceral Arousal Systems and the Pleasure-Unpleasure System are u-h-r functions, their properties should reflect certain characteristics in common, for example:

1. A capacity of each system for reciprocally antithetical equilibrium. The law of reciprocally antithetical interaction within the central nervous system characterizes states of induced autonomic sympathetic-parasympathetic imbalance. This interaction has been investigated by Gellhorn in relation to high and low blood pressure (1957:22–4;262).

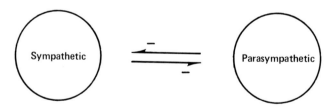

This capacity for a reciprocally antithetical equilibrium between facilitatory and inhibitory processes should also pertain to other u-h-r systems. This conclusion coincides with Hernandez-Peon's (1964:211) hypotheses that the facilitatory and inhibitory processes within the Somatic Arousal-Tranquilizing (Vigilance-Sleep) Systems and within the Pleasure-Unpleasure (Reward-Punishment) Systems are regulated by such a reciprocally antithetical interaction. The following formulae are based upon Hernandez-Peon's presentation

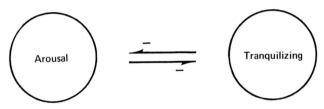

indicating that electrode stimulation within these systems would have the following effects:

⬆ AROUSAL ⟶ ⬇ TRANQUILIZING

⬇ AROUSAL ⟶ ⬆ TRANQUILIZING

⬆ TRANQUILIZING ⟶ ⬇ AROUSAL

⬇ TRANQUILIZING ⟶ ⬆ AROUSAL

⬆ = increase in the charge   Arousal = Arousal System
⬇ = decrease in the charge   Tranquilizing = Tranquilizing System

and

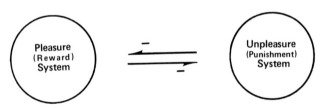

indicating that electrode stimulation within these systems should have the following effects:

⬆ PLEASURE ⟶ ⬇ UNPLEASURE

⬇ PLEASURE ⟶ ⬆ UNPLEASURE

⬆ UNPLEASURE ⟶ ⬇ PLEASURE

⬇ UNPLEASURE ⟶ ⬆ PLEASURE

⬆ = increase in the charge   Pleasure = Pleasure (Reward) System
⬇ = decrease in the charge   Unpleasure = Unpleasure (Punishment) System

2. A capacity for reverberation and prolongation of response whereby any number of differing states of arousal and tranquility, pleasure or unpleasure, or visceral excitation can be maintained over long periods of time.

3. A capacity for extensive recruitment and adaptation whereby awareness of any of these states is most pronounced when initiating stimuli are first presented and least pronounced following prolonged stimulus repetition.

4. A capacity to be charged by (a) an unconditional sensory afferent input into the reticular formation, (b) physical, metabolic, and hormonal changes affecting the hypothalamus via the blood stream, and (c) the formation of upper limbic sensory engrams which may be conditioned to innervate reactions at hypothalamic and reticular levels.

Stimulus Conditions Charging the U-H-R- Systems

Stimulus conditions charging the u-h-r systems may be analyzed in terms of a number of different parameters: (1) total energy or intensity, (2) temporal distribution (micro-frequencies determining tone and hue; also gross rate of stimulus presentation), (3) spatial distribution (including microscopic stimulus distribution, a source for texture), and (4) specificity and non-specificity or the degree of demarcated change.

Stimulus specificity refers to *demarcated stimulus change,* temporally or spatially. A sudden sound or a sudden presentation of light offers a source for temporally specific stimulation. A sharply defined pressure on the skin offers a source for spatially specific stimulation.

Specificity of stimulation may occur on a molecular or gross molar level. Stimulation of the gustatory receptors by a substance consisting of molecules of salt followed by a substance consisting of molecules of sugar, involves stimulus specificity: a demarcated change in the spatial distribution of ions, atoms, and molecules. Also, on a gross molar level, stimulation of the retina by the reflection of light from a tree and then from an automobile involves stimulus specificity: a demarcated change in spatial distribution of light energy.

Conversely, stimulus non-specificity refers to a *paucity of demarcated stimulus change,* a *high degree of stimulus constancy* temporally or spatially. For example, the high altitude aviator may be exposed for many hours to the bright light of the sky and the roaring noise of plane motors. Such stimulation is marked in an absolute sense. However, in a relative sense, it demonstrates a paucity of change temporally and spatially and therefore is non-specific.*

These concepts may further be clarified by the graphs in Fig. VII-1.

Graph A depicts extreme non-specificity of stimulation characterized by no change at all in its temporal or spatial distribution. Graph B depicts a predominance of stimulus non-specificity in that changes are not highly demarcated and no change occurs in stimulus patterns from one block of time to another. Graph C depicts extreme specificity of stimulation involving a highly demarcated, sharp, stimulus change.

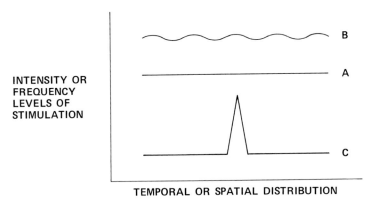

Figure VII-1. Stimulus specificity and non-specificity defined in terms of the degree of demarcated change.

* Non-specificity of stimulation, a function of paucity of demarcated change, i.e., the degree of stimulus constancy, may be measured with mathematical precision in relation to:

> constancy with no change
> constancy of rate of change
> constancy of acceleration of change

i.e., a high level of non-specificity, a high level of constancy may be maintained not only with respect to:

> change (c) = O, no change
> change (c) = k, change a constant

but also with respect to change per unit time:

$$\frac{dc}{dt} = k', \text{ rate of change a constant}$$

and

$$\frac{d^2c}{dt^2} = k'', \text{ acceleration of change a constant}$$

I

STIMULUS CONDITIONS CHARGING
THE TRANQUILIZING AND AROUSAL SYSTEMS

Stimulation Unconditionally Charging the Tranquilizing System
(presumably via the reticular formation)

Stimulation which contributes to states of tranquility and therefore assumed to be instrumental in charging the u-h-r Tranquilizing System may be shown to be characterized by:

1. *Stimulus Non-specificity:* 'Sensory deprivation' studies (Heron, 1961: 8–9, 16–17) have demonstrated that human subjects exposed primarily to unchanging, unpatterned non-specific visual, tactile, and auditory stimulation drift into a state of drowsiness, sleep, and confusion. In these studies, subjects placed in a soundproof room were exposed to (a) non-specific sound from the droning of a motor, (b) non-specific light stimulation attained through translucent glasses, and (c) non-specific tactile stimulation made possible by the use of gloves and long cardboard cuffs. Heron (1961: 16–17) notes that "the subjects preferred 'just to let their minds drift' . . . blank periods during which they could think of nothing would frequently occur . . . There were frequent reports of confusion, inability to concentrate and inability to 'think about anything to think about.' Some subjects said they were unable to distinguish between sleep and waking."

Bennett (1961:168) in his observations of aviators flying at unusually great heights reached a similar conclusion. These men who were exposed to non-specific stimulation from an unobstructed expanse of cloudless sky and from the whirling noise of airplane motors, soon lost conscious contact with surroundings and drifted into states approximating sleep.

Similarly, an infant may be lulled to sleep by being held closely in his mother's arms and gently rocked, i.e., his Tranquilizing System is charged by diffuse non-specific stimulation involving monotonous repetitive movements with little change from one block of time to another, and with little demarcated change in contact from one spatial point of the body to another (see Oswald, 1962:149–151). These findings lead to the conclusion that non-specificity of stimulation tends to charge the Tranquilizing or Sleep System.

2. *Reduced Intensity:* Low intensity of external stimulation is frequently tranquilizing. A quiet voice and gentle patting may transform an infant's state of excitement into one of normal receptivity. These effects frequently are reinforced when low intensity of stimulation is combined with non-specificity without abrupt change.

3. *Reduced Stimulus Rate:* A parallel effect is offered by a reduction in the rate of stimulation. The mother often may quiet her distraught baby by

patting him first at a rather fast rate matching the baby's on-going restless behavior and then gradually patting more and more slowly. Likewise a subject may become drowsy when a hypnotist monotonously speaks more and more slowly to him.

4. *Deep Pressure:* Deep pressure temporally and spatially non-abrupt contributes to states of tranquility. The individual who is terribly upset may be soothed by being held with firm deep pressure.° A child who is wild and screaming may be quieted by a very firm grasp of the wrist. Two frightened people may cling to one another and in this way become comforted and pacified.

Stimulation Unconditionally Charging the Arousal System (presumably via the reticular formation)

The stimulus characteristics associated with charging the Arousal System should be the opposite of those associated with charging the Tranquilizing System: (1) temporal and spatial specificity, (2) marked intensity, (3) increasing rate, and (4) superficial versus deep tactile application.

1. *Stimulus Specificity:* A poke involves a sharply demarcated, highly specific stimulus. Frequently it eventuates in heightened states of arousal and when repeated may lead to a discharge of excitement with outbursts of laughter or aggression.

"Sharp," highly demarcated noises, tastes, or colors also are obvious sources for elevated states of arousal.

2. *High intensity:* A relation between increasing intensity of stimulation and elevated charge of the non-specific Arousal System hardly needs elaboration. Screaming and yelling, bright lights, and heavy handling regularly contribute to mounting excitement.

3. *Increasing Rate of Stimulation:* The quickening beat of the drum during tribal battle, a mounting rate of applause at a rally, or the wild speed of the auto races offer examples of the relation between the increasing rate of stimulation and the charging of states of heightened arousal.

4. *Light Tactile Touch:* Light touch when specifically applied to the superficial sensory receptors offers a basis for charging the Arousal System. Touch which contacts the upper surface of the hair follicles without affecting the deep pressure receptors, for example, is a primary component of tickling that in turn activates mounting arousal and excitement.

Table XI presents in outline form a summary of these conditions which have been suggested as possible sources for charging the Arousal and Tranquilizing Systems.

° To be differentiated from restriction of behavior.

TABLE XI
STIMULUS CONDITIONS CHARGING THE AROUSAL AND
TRANQUILIZING SYSTEMS

Charging the Arousal System	Charging the Tranquilizing System
1. Specificity of stimulation characterized by demarcated change, abruptness	1. Non-specificity of stimulation characterized by a paucity of demarcated change
2. Increasing intensity of stimulation	2. Decreasing intensity of stimulation
3. Increasing rate of stimulation	3. Decreasing rate of stimulation
4. Innervation of the superficial erogenous sensory receptors	4. Innervation of the deep pressure sensory receptors

II

STIMULUS CONDITIONS CHARGING THE UNPLEASURE AND PLEASURE SYSTEMS

Stimulation Unconditionally Charging the Unpleasure System

The following stimulus conditions regularly elicit unpleasurable states (presumably via a sensory input into the reticular formation) and are therefore assumed to serve as sources for charging the Unpleasure-Punishment System.

1. *Pain Stimulation:* Stimulus conditions eliciting pain are regularly recognized as a source of punishment and unpleasurable emotion. In the language of activation theory, pain innervation may be said to be a source for charging the non-specific Unpleasure System.

Sweet (1959:459–502) points out that pain stimulation primarily involves the penetration of tissues containing the free-nerve-ending pain receptors. This process may result from mechanical penetration of the skin, intense heat, electric stimulation, distention of the viscera, excessive arterio-dilatation, ischemia associated with arterio-constriction, and inflammation of body tissues. Frequently these processes involve high intensity and extreme specificity, i.e., sharpness characterizing stimulation of the sensory receptors.

2. *Gustatory Stimulation:* Concentrated stimulation of the sour, salt, and bitter taste receptors will regularly elicit unpleasurable feelings (see Pfaffman, 1959:529–30). Stimulation of these taste receptors therefore can provide another source for charging the Unpleasure System. Figure VII–2 illustrates these findings.

The characteristics of stimuli which can innervate these taste receptors (ibid:513–22) are related on a molecular level to the specific spatial distribution of substances applied to the tongue. For example, Figure VII–3 from Pfaffman's report illustrates how the spatial arangement of $-NO_2$, $-CH_3$ and $-NH_2$ radicals of a given compound may determine whether bitter or sweet taste receptors become innervated during gustatory contact and therefore whether or not the Unpleasure System is activated. Since the solitary nucleus mediating the sensory aspects of taste is embedded within the reticular formation, innervation of this nucleus by impulses from the taste receptors is in a position to affect reticular patterns of non-specific pleasure and unpleasure activation.

3. *Excessive Arousal Stimulation:* Evidence has been presented to the effect that general arousal and pleasure-unpleasure are partially indepen-

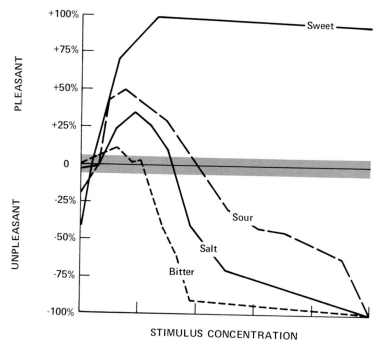

EAG

Figure VII-2. "Preponderance of pleasant or unpleasant judgments in relation to the concentration of solution tasted. The ordinate gives percent pleasant minus percent unpleasant. The abscissa is proportional to the concentration: the full length of the line standing for 40% cane sugar, 1.12% tartaric acid, 10% NaCl, and 0.004% quinine sulfate (all by weight)." (Adapted from Woodworth's reproduction of Engel, R., in Woodworth, R.S., Ed.: *Experimental Psychology.* New York: Holt, 1938, p. 498.)

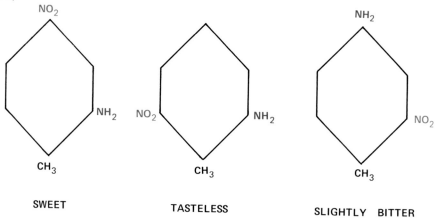

EAG

Figure VII-3. Specific spatial molecular arrangement as a determinant of taste. (Redrawn with permission, from Pfaffman, C.: The sense of taste. In Field, J., Magoun, H.W., and Hall, V., Eds.: *Handbook of Physiology, Section on Neurophysiology,* Vol. I. Washington, D.C.: Am Physiological Soc, 1959, p. 519.)

dent, partially dependent° functions. According to this theoretical formulation, conditions charging the Arousal System, e.g., marked stimulus intensity and specificity, should be in a position to affect the charge of the Pleasure and Unpleasure Systems. There appears to exist for each individual at a given time an upper threshold which determines the level of arousal stimulation *above* which the Unpleasure System becomes charged. When such an arousal-unpleasure threshold is low, then stimulation of even moderate intensity and specific abruptness would tend to activate states of unpleasure. Poking, tickling, and bouncing, which early in the day evoke a toddler's expressions of glee and laughter, elicit states of unpleasure at the end of his long day when his arousal-unpleasure threshold is low.

An arousal-unpleasure threshold would be expected to differ not only from one moment of the day to another for a given individual, but also from one individual to another. Some people may be able to tolerate massive stimulus arousal conditions: long periods of loud, sharp, sudden noises, bright lights, shoving and pushing; for others, these stimulus conditions frequently precipitate states of marked unpleasure.

4. *Deficient Arousal Stimulation:* Conversely, a deficiency of demarcated change or novelty (a deficiency of stimulus specificity) leads to states of "boredom" and discontent. In the language of non-specific activation theory, a deficiency of arousal stimulation tends to charge the non-specific Unpleasure System. According to this concept, there exists for a given individual at a given time a second threshold of arousal stimulation *below* which the non-specific Unpleasure System is charged.

A demonstration of a deficiency of arousal stimulation as a source for charging the Unpleasure System is offered by Ribble's studies of sensory deprivation during infancy (1965:4–12). These studies indicate that infants exposed to excessively insufficient arousal develop a state of depressive "marasmus."

5. *Interruption of Conditions Charging The Pleasure System:* If reduction of *electrode* charge of the Pleasure System results in an increment in the charge of the antithetical Unpleasure System, then a reduction or interruption of *external conditions* charging the Pleasure System should also result in an increment in the charge of the Unpleasure System.

This hypothesis is amply illustrated by clinical studies of "emotional loss" involving the interruption, temporary or prolonged, of conditions which were contributing to pleasure states. An infant or child may encounter loss of his mother's presence, loss of his blanket or soft teddy bear, or may become preoccupied with concerns of loss or damage to a part of his body.

° They are dependent to the extent that they are functions of reticular non-specific activation.

In these cases even a temporary interruption or loss of pleasure-producing conditions will evoke unpleasure in the form of anger, grief, anxiety, or depression. In terms of activation theory, interruption of conditions which were in the process of charging the Pleasure System eventuates in the charging of the antithetical Unpleasure System.

6. *Interruption of Discharge of Innervated Response*: Interruption or blocking of innervated *response*, a concept to be differentiated from interruption of *stimulus* conditions charging the Pleasure System, has been studied both clinically and experimentally. Such investigation indicates that muscular restriction interrupting the discharge of innervated reactions contributes to the charging of unpleasure states. Tseng (1942; see Arnold, 1960:225) found that a dual operation of poking rats with straws together with restriction of discharge of response, evoked violent anger. Psychoanalysts who have studied infants and children, also conclude that restriction of behavioral discharge elicits unpleasure. Mittelman (1954: 161) notes that "in the first year of life . . . chiefly restriction, e.g., during diapering or being dressed, and interference with activities . . . produce chiefly rage. . . ." Hartmann, Kris, and Lowenstein (1949:30) refer to the well-known observation that "any interruption of activity, at least in the child, is likely to evoke an aggressive response; . . . non-completion of actions specifically affects aggression . . . the child without outlet tends to be naughty."

The physiological bases upon which these effects are determined have not as yet been investigated. One wonders if they are not associated with muscular tension resulting from restriction of muscular contraction. Such tension may prove to be associated with the degree of tautness of the intrafusial muscles. Current neurophysiological experimental findings point to the prominent part played by these muscle strands, the intrafusial fibres, within the internal connective tissues of each muscle (see Ruch, 1965:199–203). Contraction of intrafusial fibres adds significantly to the afferent discharge of the spindle. Figure VII–4 indicates how the restriction of innervated muscle contraction eventuates in an increase of intrafusial tension. Proprioceptive impulses arising from muscle tension are relayed to the cerebellum and from there to the reticular system (see Brookhart, 1960: 1252, 1249). Connections with the reticular formation therefore provide a possible route by which muscular tension, like pain or excessive arousal stimulation, may charge the Unpleasure System.

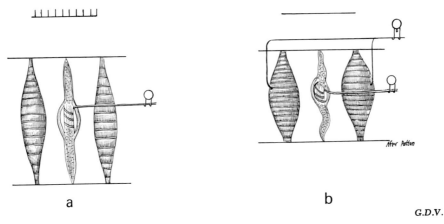

Figure VII-4. (a) Intrafusial muscle tension is elevated when innervated muscle contraction is restricted. (b) Intrafusial muscle tension is reduced during innervated muscle contraction. (Redrawn with permission, from Patton, H.: Reflex regulation of movement and posture. In Ruch, T., Patton, H., Woodbury, J., and Towe, A.: *Neurophysiology*, 2nd ed. Philadelphia: Saunders, 1965, p. 190.)

Stimulation Unconditionally Charging the Pleasure System

The following stimulus conditions regularly elicit states of pleasure (presumably via a sensory input into the reticular formation) and are therefore assumed to serve as sources for charging the Pleasure-Reward System.

1. *Erogenous Stimulation:* Tactile contact with the erogenous areas of the skin is a commonly accepted source for reactions of pleasure.

2. *Gustatory Stimulation:* Stimulation of the taste receptors for "sweetness" as well as limited stimulation of the "salt," "bitter," or "sour" taste receptors (a function of the spatial distribution of atoms and molecules of substances in contact with the tongue) offer another source for pleasure (see Figs. VII–2 and VII–3).

3. *A Modicum of Arousal Stimulation:* The introduction of a limited amount of arousal stimulation, during a deficiency of arousal stimulation, should charge the Pleasure System. For example, when a non-specific monotonous day-to-day routine provides a basis for a deficiency of arousal stimulation, the introduction of excitement or any novel demarcated change as a source for arousal comes as a pleasurable relief: a trip to new lands, a new job, a new set of decorations for the house, or even a quarrel.

4. *A Modicum of Tranquilizing Stimulation:* During excessive arousal, the application of comforting, tranquilizing stimulation has been known to afford pleasurable relief. The infant who has begun to cry and scream after visitors have treated him too noisily and roughly may require non-specific stimulation: gentle rocking and tender patting before he can be restored to a state of peaceful contentment.

5. *The Interruption of Unpleasurable Stimulus Conditions:* According to the formulation that there exists a reciprocally antithetical relation between the charges of the Pleasure and Unpleasure Systems, the interruption or removal of external conditions which were in the process of charging the Unpleasure System should reciprocally charge the Pleasure System:

$$\downarrow \text{Unpl} \longrightarrow \uparrow \text{Pl}$$

Actual experience confirms this conclusion. The removal of discomfort from pain or from bowel or bladder tension offers pleasurable relief; so does the removal of an unpleasant guest or a disturbing defect.

6. *Release from Muscular Restriction:* If heightened intrafusial muscle tension during restriction of innervated muscle contraction contributes to elevation of Unpleasure System charge, then release of innervated muscle response with a reduction of intrafusial tension (see Fig. VII–4) should result in a reciprocally antithetical charge of the Pleasure System. Particularly among children or adults who have not learned to accept controls, restrictions and waiting are poorly tolerated, whereas freedom from restriction is pleasurable. This conclusion has been emphasized in Freud's Pleasure Principle which states that since the direct relief of tension is pleasurable, mankind often finds it difficult to accept restrictions and to tolerate postponement (Freud, 1955:7, 10; Aichhorn, 1935:191–8). Hartmann, Kris, and Lowenstein (1949:27) conclude that even the direct discharge of aggressive behavior is pleasurable, a possible reason for the unrelenting persistence of warfare throughout the history of the human race.

Table XII presents in outline form conditions which have been suggested as possible sources for charging the Pleasure (Reward) and Unpleasure (Punishment) Systems. The table also includes reference to chemical and physical changes within the bloodstream and to the conditioning of neutral stimuli, as sources for charging these systems.

TABLE XII
STIMULUS CONDITIONS CHARGING THE PLEASURE AND UNPLEASURE SYSTEMS

Charging the Unpleasure System	Charging the Pleasure System
1. Pain stimulation (via the reticular formation)	1. Erotogenic stimulation (presumably via the reticular formation)
2. Bitter and sour (concentrated) gustatory stimulation (presumably via the reticular formation)	2. Sweet gustatory stimulation (presumably via the reticular formation)
3. Metabolic conditions within the bloodstream during hunger, thirst, and during excessive or deficient thermal stimulation (via the hypothalamus)	3. Metabolic conditions within the bloodstream during satiation of hunger and thirst; moderate thermal stimulation (via the hypothalamus)
4. Conditional stimulus activation of unpleasure (presumably via upper limbic areas)	4. Conditional stimulus activation of pleasure (presumably via upper limbic areas)
5. Excess arousal stimulation	5. A modicum of tranquilizing stimulation inhibiting excessive arousal
6. Deficient arousal stimulation	6. A modicum of arousal stimulation during a deficiency of arousal stimulation
7. Interruption of Pleasure System charge	7. Interruption of Unpleasure System charge
8. Tension due to restriction of innervated response (via reticular formation)	8. Tension reduction due to discharge of innervated response (via reticular formation)

Chapter VIII

A U-H-R Activation Theory of Emotion

The Somatic Arousal, Pleasure and Unpleasure, and Visceral Arousal Systems have been defined as behavioral systems whose properties are derivatives of the following forms of u-h-r system circuit discharge (see Fig. VI–3):

1. Ascending tonic and phasic non-specific arousal activation.
2. Ascending patterns of phasic non-specific pleasure and unpleasure activation.
3. Descending tonic non-specific activation.
4. Descending extrapyramidal rhythmic reactions.
5. Sympathetic and parasympathetic visceral activation.
6. Pituitary endocrine activation.

It is proposed that emotion consists of combinations of behavioral and perceptual reactions related to these six forms of u-h-r system discharge which become expressed psychologically in the form of the following states:

1. *Excitement*, its presence or absence, a function of all six avenues of u-h-r system discharge determining excitable, agitated, calm, or apathetic feelings.

2. *Muscular tension and relaxation*, a function of u-h-r system discharge via descending non-specific activation affecting muscular tonus, general bodily stance and facial cast, and contributing under stress to muscular tenseness and spasm.

3. The release of *rhythmic movements*, a function of u-h-r discharge via extrapyramidal reactions determining states which range from hyperactivity and restlessness to placidity and inertia.

4. *Pleasure* or *unpleasure*, a function of u-h-r system discharge via patterns of ascending phasic non-specific activation, determining feelings of "cheer," "joy," "sorrow," and "discontent."

5. *Psychosomatic visceral reactions*, a function of u-h-r system discharge via autonomic and pituitary endocrine activation.

Table XIII presents an analysis of anger, fear, grief, depression, and joy in terms of these non-specific physiological reactions and their psychological correlates:

TABLE XIII
AN ANALYSIS OF EMOTION IN TERMS OF NON-SPECIFIC NEUROPHYSIOLOGICAL REACTIONS AND THEIR PSYCHOLOGICAL CORRELATES

(read vertically)

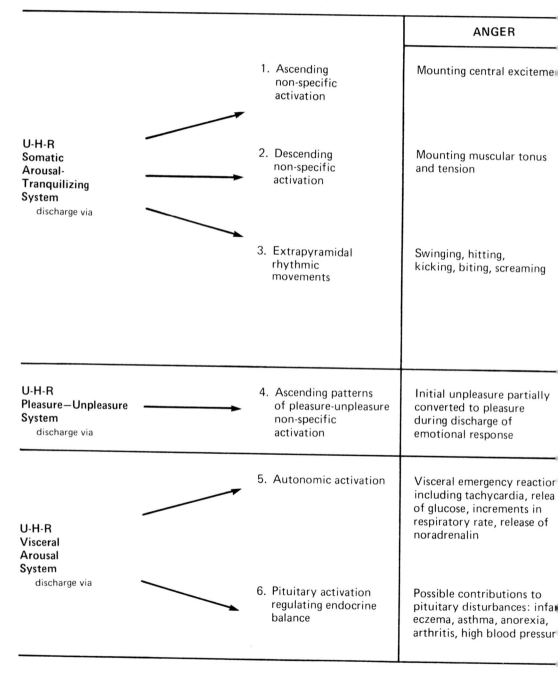

		ANGER
U-H-R Somatic Arousal-Tranquilizing System discharge via	1. Ascending non-specific activation	Mounting central exciteme
	2. Descending non-specific activation	Mounting muscular tonus and tension
	3. Extrapyramidal rhythmic movements	Swinging, hitting, kicking, biting, screaming
U-H-R Pleasure—Unpleasure System discharge via	4. Ascending patterns of pleasure-unpleasure non-specific activation	Initial unpleasure partially converted to pleasure during discharge of emotional response
U-H-R Visceral Arousal System discharge via	5. Autonomic activation	Visceral emergency reaction including tachycardia, relea of glucose, increments in respiratory rate, release of noradrenalin
	6. Pituitary activation regulating endocrine balance	Possible contributions to pituitary disturbances: infa eczema, asthma, anorexia, arthritis, high blood pressur

FEAR	GRIEF	DEPRESSION	JOY
ting central ment often to oint of complete r and perceptual ganization	Reduced alertness	Inhibition of central excitation with clouded consciousness and a tendency toward withdrawal into sleep	Optimal levels of central excitement
ting muscular n often to the of immobilization uscular collapse	Loss of tonicity affecting the anti-gravity musculature and associated with fallen cast of face, head and shoulders, stumbling and collapse	Markedly decreased muscular tone; in extreme cases among infants, muscular collapse	Optimal levels of muscular tonus; uplifted facial cast and bodily stance
ng movements of ody, head, and a basis for avoid- adduction and n of limbs, a basis ithdrawal and ing; arrest reactions, obilization	General inhibition of activity; slowness of pace, sobbing respiratory movements	Marked inhibition of activity	Release of rhythmic reactions, an integral part of play response: rolling, tumbling, jumping, flapping, etc.
ed unrelieved easure	Marked unpleasure	Marked unpleasure	Marked pleasure
eral emergency tions with the se of adrenalin	Parasympathetic discharge with shedding of tears	Inhibition of sympathetic and parasympathetic discharge with absence of tears and loss of appetite; constipation, urinary retention, sexual dysfunction Possible trophic dis-turbances in ACTH regulation with in-creased susceptibility to disease	Optimal viscero-tonic background for nonstressful activity

Chapter IX

The Organization of
Sexual and Maternal Behavior

In this chapter, sexual and maternal behavior will be analyzed in terms of both *specific* sensory-motor response constellations and *non-specific* "emotional" and "motivational" processes.

I

THE U-H-R SEXUAL SYSTEM

The Discharge of Sexual Behavior

Organization of Sexual Behavior at Reticular, Hypothalamic, and Upper Limbic Levels

Reticular processes mediate fragmented sexual reactions. For example, spawning movements of the frog are organized within the brainstem tegmentum i.e. reticular formation (see review by Beach, 1951:399). Experimental studies among primates (MacLean and Denniston, 1963:281–3) have shown that loci for penile erection are found along the medial forebrain bundle within the ventral and lateral reticular formation of the midbrain and pons; additionally loci for seminal discharge and genital scratching are present within the medial thalamic reticular areas (MacLean, 1962:295; MacLean and Ploog, 1962:52). The neural organization of sexual behavior, however, occurs primarily within the *hypothalamus*. Both Sawyer (1960: 1225–38) and Grossman (1967:467–78) present extensive reviews of experimental studies which indicate that areas predominantly within (1) the posterior hypothalamus activate the sexual hormones of the pituitary via the hypothalamic-hypophysial portal system (see Chapter VI); and (2) areas in the region of the anterior hypothalamus regulate rhythmic patterns of sexual behavior, e.g., via the medial forebrain bundle terminating within the reticular formation. Lesions of the anterior hypothalamus result in the permanent disappearance of organized sexual behavior even though sexual hormones are maintained at adequate levels. Additionally, implanted electrode studies demonstrate that sexual stimulation of the vagina results in EEG changes localized within the anterior hypothalamus.

Upper limbic contributions to sexual behavior also have been reported.

91

MacLean (1963:21–2) has shown that electrode stimulation of the hippo-campus and septal nuclei elicits sexual grooming behavior, while stimulation of the hippocampus, septal nuclei, and cingulate cortex activates penile erection. Kluver and Bucy (1939:992) have demonstrated that hypersexual behavior which involves oral and visual preoccupations results from lesions of the amygdala and of the pyriform and temporal cortices. Delgado (1969: 144–5) has described complex sexual reaction elicited by electrode stimulation of the upper limbic temporal cortex. One of his patients, a 36-year-old female, who was undergoing implanted electrode studies, reported that when the right temporal lobe was stimulated she felt "a pleasant tingling sensation in the left side of her body 'from my face down to the bottom of my legs.' She started giggling . . . stating that she enjoyed the sensation 'very much.' Repetition of these stimulations made the patient more . . . flirtatious and she ended by openly expressing her desire to marry the therapist. Stimulation of other cerebral points failed to modify her mood. . . . During control interviews before and after electrical stimulation of the brain, her behavior was quite proper without familiarity . . . ." Likewise it has been shown that among human patients prefrontal lesions eventuate in sexual disinhibition (see Brutkowski, 1964:244–5).

The upper limbic, hypothalamic, and reticular organization of sexual behavior presumably pertains not only to specific but also to non-specific reactions. According to this conclusion, sexual emotion like other emotions would be understood to be a function of u-h-r system discharge via six avenues of non-specific activation. A tentative analysis of sexual emotion in these terms is presented in Table XIV.

Processes by Which the
Sexual System May Be Charged

On the basis that the processes of the u-h-r Sexual System would be expected to reflect the characteristics of u-h-r systems in general, it is proposed that stimulus conditions may charge the Sexual System via three principal routes: (1) an extrinsic unconditional tactile-erotogenic input into the reticular formation, (2) an unconditional chemical-hormonal hypo-thalamic input, and (3) a conditional (e.g. visual) input determining the formation of intrinsic upper limbic engrams which may become associated with hypothalamic-reticular patterns of sexual reaction. Since tactile-erotogenic, hormonal, and visual erotic stimulation may be shown to serve as the principal sources for sexual arousal in man, the considerations to follow will focus upon these stimulus conditions.

Tactile-Erotogenic Stimulation

Tactile stimulation of the erotogenic zones of the body provides an

TABLE XIV
SEXUAL EMOTION
(read vertically)

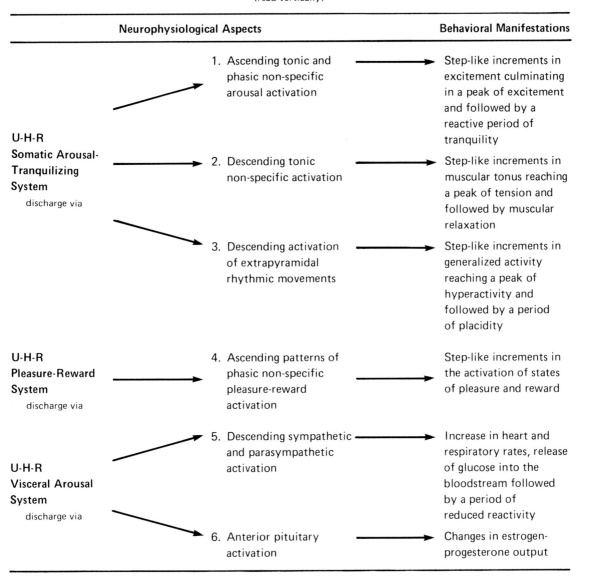

Neurophysiological Aspects	Behavioral Manifestations
U-H-R Somatic Arousal-Tranquilizing System discharge via	
1. Ascending tonic and phasic non-specific arousal activation	Step-like increments in excitement culminating in a peak of excitement and followed by a reactive period of tranquility
2. Descending tonic non-specific activation	Step-like increments in muscular tonus reaching a peak of tension and followed by muscular relaxation
3. Descending activation of extrapyramidal rhythmic movements	Step-like increments in generalized activity reaching a peak of hyperactivity and followed by a period of placidity
U-H-R Pleasure-Reward System discharge via	
4. Ascending patterns of phasic non-specific pleasure-reward activation	Step-like increments in the activation of states of pleasure and reward
U-H-R Visceral Arousal System discharge via	
5. Descending sympathetic and parasympathetic activation	Increase in heart and respiratory rates, release of glucose into the bloodstream followed by a period of reduced reactivity
6. Anterior pituitary activation	Changes in estrogen-progesterone output

TABLE XV
TACTILE STIMULATION AS A SOURCE FOR SEXUAL AROUSAL

Order	Tactile Stimulation	Sexual Behavior
Amphibia: leopard frog	Tactile stimulation of the female from clasp by the male	Spawning movements
	Simultaneous tactile stimulation of the male from female contractions as she expels her eggs	Ejaculatory pumping
Reptiles: lizard	Tactile stimulation of the female as the male holds her neck in his jaw or bites other portions of her body	Copulatory cooperation
	Tactile stimulation of the female from the combs of the male's thighs	Copulatory cooperation
Mammals: rat	Stimulation of the oestrous female from palpation or stroking of her back or sides, e.g., by the experimenter	Mating responses
hamster, porcupine, skunk, dog	Tactile stimulation of the female from the male's licking, nibbling or scratching her vaginal region	Maintenance of mating posture
cat	Stimulation of the oestrous female from gripping loose skin of her neck with pressure on her back	Mating posture

essential source for unconditional activation of sexual arousal. Beach (1951: 394–8) cites pertinent findings from the experimental literature with respect to studies carried out among a wide variety of orders and species. Typical findings are summarized in Table XV.

Among humans, the role of tactile stimulation of the erogenous mucous membranes in relation to sexual arousal is generally accepted knowledge.

Hormonal Conditions

Elevation in the blood level content of the sexual hormones activates sexual mating behavior. These effects are produced not only by the secretory activity of the ovaries or testes at puberty but also by the injection of estrogens or androgens in immature animal subjects (Beach, 1942:285–92).

An endocrine feedback process operates between the hypothalamus and the sexual glands (Szentagothai, 1962; see also Davidson, 1966:584–98; Urquhart, 1971:227): hypothalamic discharge to the anterior pituitary activates the secretion of the gonadotrophic hormones into the bloodstream, a basis for stimulation of ovarian and testicular secretion of estrogen, progesterone, and testosterone. Vascular distribution of the sexual hormones back to the hypothalamus completes the cycle by dampening further hypothalamic-pituitary activation of the gonadotrophic hormones. The action of the sexual hormones upon the hypothalamic receptors provide also a most likely source for sexual hormone charge of the Sexual System circuits and for oestrous manifestations of Sexual System discharge via heightened levels of activity and sexual receptivity.

Visual Stimulation

Although olfaction has been considered a primary source for sexual arousal among many quadrupeds (Beach, 1951:396), visual stimulation tends to replace olfaction among animals whose modus vivendi provides for less olfactory contact with the ground, e. g., among birds and primates including man. The role of vision in human sexuality is reflected by the frequency with which visual attention to the body and its movements contributes to sexual forepleasure culminating in sexual intercourse.*

Vision actually exerts important effects upon sexual arousal not only among primates but also among most lower animal forms including fish, amphibia, reptiles, and birds. This conclusion derives from findings reported in the experimental literature as reviewed by Beach (ibid:392–6). Table XVI outlines some of these findings.

Subcortical upper limbic structures presumably mediate such visual contributions to sexual arousal. This conclusion is suggested by Kluver and

---

* It is also reflected by the deluge of pornographic display in our present society. "Erotica" has become the synonym for a visual absorption with the genitalia and related erogenous zones.

TABLE XVI
VISUAL STIMULATION AS A SOURCE FOR SEXUAL AROUSAL

Order	Tactile Stimulation	Sexual Behavior
Fish: male stickelback	The male's observation of the swollen abdomen of a female fish model	Sexual arousal
Amphibia: frog	No visual stimulation (blinded subjects)	No sexual approach
Reptiles: female lizard	The female's observation of the male's extending dewlaps and bobbing head up and down	Sexual receptivity
Birds: male pheasant	The male's observation of stuffed skin of a female pheasant	Copulatory behavior
robin	The male's observation of mounted bird with red breast	(Aggression)
	The male's observation of mounted bird lacking a red breast	Copulatory behavior

Bucy's findings (1939:992) that bilateral lobectomy of the upper limbic temporal and pyriform cortices and a portion of the amygdala releases an exaggerated hypersexuality which involves visual preoccupations.

Stimulus Conditioning

Beach (1951:408–10) reviews numerous experimental studies which indicate that sexual behavior may be conditioned. With respect to inhibitory effects, for example, male rats who have received electric shock during or immediately after copulation with receptive females usually fail to mate when they are reintroduced into the testing stimulus situation. Conversely, initially neutral stimuli may be positively conditioned to activate sexual arousal mechanisms. Beach (ibid: 409) notes that "male rats that have copulated with receptive females in a particular cage often attempt to mate with males or non-receptive females encountered in the original testing situation." Breder and Coates (1935:187–207) demonstrated that neutral stimuli may be conditioned to elicit sexual arousal among fish. In one experiment, male guppies were placed in a tank where they were able to swim freely. Then a glass beaker containing water was suspended within the tank. The male guppies showed no signs of sexual arousal in the presence of the suspended beaker. Next the beaker was removed and then with a receptive female enclosed, it was reintroduced into the male fish tank. The presentation of the beaker with its enclosed content was repeated at hourly intervals. On each occasion the male guppies were sexually aroused. Finally an empty beaker was once again lowered into the male tank. This time the initially neutral visual stimulus evoked sexual attempts of the male fish.

The areas of the central nervous system that mediate these conditional associations have not yet been determined. The present u-h-r non-specific activation theory of sexual emotion suggests that upper limbic areas provide for the formation of sensory engrams which may become associated with hypothalamic-reticular patterns of sexual activation. This hypothesis may be directly tested by experiments which measure the degree to which an animal's capacity for sexual conditioning is impaired by lesions of specific upper limbic foci.

Visual Stimulation and Sexual Imprinting

Among lower forms of animal life, sexual responsiveness to the visual characteristics of a mate (see Table XVI) does not usually differ from one subject to another for a given species. Therefore, it is assumed that these reactions are determined by a constitutional predilection or result from a common experience to which all members of a specific species are equally exposed. Konrad Lorenz's findings (1957:102–10) with respect to sexual imprinting favor the latter explanation.

Sexual imprinting, most obvious among birds, involves the formation of visual representations during the neonatal period. Whomever the baby bird sees during an early critical period of life sets the visual pattern which later will evoke its sexual responses. If it happens to be a human being who is seen, it will only be a human being to which this bird becomes sexually attracted during his years of sexual maturity.

Neurophysiological mechanisms which mediate sexual imprinting have not as yet been discovered, but information which has been presented in this chapter in relation to upper limbic, hypothalamic, and reticular contributions to sexual behavior suggests a u-h-r theory of sexual imprinting. According to such a theory, sexual imprinting would involve the association of a specific visual contact with on-going processes of the Pleasure-Reward System (e.g. activated via hormonal, metabolic, proprioceptive, or arousal stimulation).° Similarly, imprinting-like processes among mammals may prove to be a function of the following variables:

1. Visual stimulus presentation of the mother to the newborn.

2. Concomitant unconditional charging of the newborn's Pleasure-Reward System during the mother's care and administration, i.e., derived from (a) reduction of unpleasure states of hunger, thirst, and cold, and (b) tactile and thermal stimulation from the mother's soft warm body.

3. Some minimal charge of the infant's Sexual System in response to maternal, tactile stimulation of its erogenous sensory receptors after birth.† With low sexual hormone levels during infancy, stimulation would still be expected to charge the Sexual System circuits, but discharge would be greatly reduced (Beach, 1942:290). Sexual imprinting in such a case would be understood to be an equivalent of early irreversible sexual conditioning as indicated by the schematization in Figure IX–1.

According to the schematization presented in Figure IX–1, sexual imprinting depends upon the association early in life of an upper limbic representation of a species member with the processes of the Pleasure-Reward and Sexual Systems. With an elevation of sexual hormone levels at puberty the same representation should evoke overt discharge of the Sexual as well as the Pleasure-Reward Systems. This theory should be able to be investigated directly. Experiments, for example, could test whether (1) early tactile stimulation and concomitant visual contact with a "parent" and (2) intactness of specific upper limbic areas (e.g., the septal nuclei, the hippocampal nuclei) are essential for the development of sexual imprinting as an

---

° Pleasure-reward reinforcement of sensory contacts is considered in Chapter XI.

† The Sexual System is intact at birth: Boling (1939:128–32) notes that for a few hours after birth while hormonal levels of the infant's bloodstream are still high as the result of the previous interconnection with the mother's bloodstream, infant guinea pigs respond to tactile stimulation of the perineal region by adopting the mating posture of the adult female.

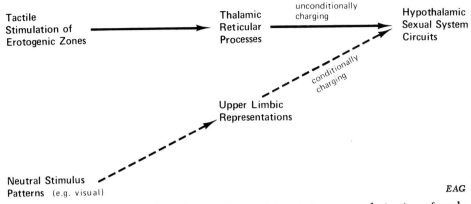

Figure IX-1. A theoretical formulation of sexual imprinting as a derivative of early irreversible conditioning.

equivalent of irreversible conditioning.*

Harlow's (1962:136–46) experiments on monkeys reared by cage-surrogate mothers suggest that primates are vulnerable to early sexual imprinting-like processes which eventuate in irreversible effects upon their adult sexual behavior. In these experiments, the infant monkey-subjects received milk and warmth from an artificial cage mother (see Fig. IX–2). There was no early opportunity for the simultaneous presentation of visual and tactile-erotogenic contact with a living monkey and therefore no opportunity for the representations of a living monkey to be associated with the Reward and Sexual Systems. Upon reaching puberty these monkeys would be lacking the early experience which would make possible positive attraction† and sexual arousal in the presence of a receptive partner. Harlow's findings support this conclusion: his experimental monkeys who lacked early visual tactile species contacts did fail at the time of maturity to react sexually to even the most receptive species members.

With respect to imprinting-like processes among humans, the part played by earliest experiences in the establishment of a capacity for adult sexual responsiveness has been studied by Greenacre. According to Greenacre, (1953:89–90) deprivation of human contacts during infancy contributes to

---

* If sexual imprinting involves upper limbic innervation concomitantly with Sexual System activation, the neurophysiological processes taking place may pertain not to the establishment of *connections* between an upper limbic trace and the Sexual System, but rather the establishment of a *trace* within an upper limbic area at a point which from the start is connected with the Sexual System. This theory of imprinting suggests the possibility that conditioning in general may involve not the establishment of connections between traces, but rather the establishment of traces at connected neural points, i.e. during concomitant innervation of these connected neural points.

† The relation of positive attraction to pleasure-reward activation is considered in Chapter XI.

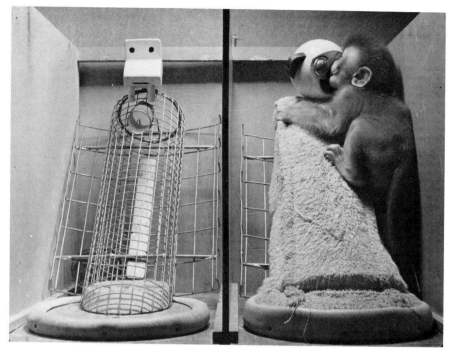

Figure IX-2. Wire and cloth-covered "mothers" used in experiments by Harlow. (Reproduced with permission, from Harlow, H.: The nature of love. *Am Psychol, 13:*673, 1958.)

subsequent difficulties with respect to sexual arousal. Like the Harlow monkeys, Greenacre's patients failed to react adequately with their own species members; rather they tended to react sexually to visual and tactile contact with inanimate objects (in the form of sexual fetishism).

Experiential processes as a source for sexual arousal among primates and man have been shown to be less rigid than among birds and lower forms of animal life; there develops an increasing flexibility in the number of stimulus associations which may be formed and in the length of time during which these associations can be modified (Beach, 1958:278–9). This increased flexibility with respect to sexual emotional conditioning coincides with an extensive development of the upper limbic system and its neocortical derivatives.

In summary, it has been shown that complex manifestations of sexual behavior are functions of upper limbic, hypothalamic, and reticular processes presumably via the discharge of the u-h-r sexual system circuits. Attention has been directed to processes by which these circuits may be charged in relation to erogenous-tactile, hormonal, and visual stimulus conditions.

II

THE U-H-R MATERNAL SYSTEM

The Discharge of Maternal Behavior

The Organization of Maternal Behavior at Hypothalamic and Upper Limbic Levels

Hypothalamic discharge via the hypophysial portal system has been found to affect the output of prolactin, the anterior pituitary hormone regulating the growth of the mammary glands and their *production of milk* (Meites, 1966:688–90). Additionally, neural pathways containing approximately 100,000 fibres in man (Rasmussen, 1940:245) descend from the hypothalamus to the posterior lobe of the pituitary gland (see Fig. VI–2). Via this route, hypothalamic stimulation activates the posterior pituitary secretion of oxytocin. The vascular distribution of this hormone to the mammary glands regulates the *ejection of milk.* Cross and Harris (1952:148) found that among rabbits electrical stimulation of the tracts running from the supraoptic nucleus of the hypothalamus to the posterior pituitary gland evokes milk ejection from a cannulated teat duct. Andersson (see Harris, 1960:1032) demonstrated the same findings with respect to unanesthetized sheep and goats. These effects of hypothalamic stimulation were shown to be mediated via the vascular transmission of posterior pituitary hormones to the mammary gland rather than via efferent tracts to these glands: denervation of the udder did not affect the results but injection of blood from another hypothalamically stimulated animal did increase milk ejection.

Upper limbic contributions to the discharge of the specific components of maternal behavior have been described by Stamm (1955:347), who found that relatively small lesions in the cingulate cortex interfere very seriously with litter survival, nest building and repair, retrieving the young and removing them from excessive heat.

The organization of these specific components of maternal behavior at hypothalamic and upper limbic levels suggests a u-h-r theory of maternal behavior and emotion. Maternal emotion like other emotions would be understood to be a function of u-h-r discharge via six avenues of non-specific activation. An analysis of maternal emotion in these terms is presented in Table XVII.

TABLE XVII
MATERNAL EMOTION

(read vertically)

Neurophysiological Aspects		Behavioral Manifestations
U-H-R Tranquilizing System discharge inhibiting	1. Ascending tonic and phasic non-specific activation	Reduced levels of excitement
	2. Descending tonic non-specific activation	Muscular relaxation; diminished forcefulness and gentleness
	3. Descending activation of extrapyramidal rhythmic movements	Reduction of hyperactivity providing for states of placidity
U-H-R Pleasure-Reward System discharge via	4. Ascending patterns of phasic non-specific activation	A generalized state of reward and pleasure
U-H-R °Visceral Arousal System discharge via	5. Descending non-specific autonomic visceral activation	Increase in nutritive functions; increased blood flow to the skin providing for the irradiation of warmth
	6. Activation of pituitary secretion of prolactin and oxytocin	The mammary flow of milk

° Trophotrophic—Parasympathetic division.

Stimulus Conditions Charging
the Maternal System

The u-h-r Maternal System, like other u-h-r systems, it is proposed, may be charged via (1) an extrinsic unconditional input into the reticular formation from sensory contacts, (2) an unconditional hormonal hypothalamic input, and (3) a conditional sensory input determining the formation of upper limbic sensory engrams that may become associated with hypothalamic-reticular patterns of maternal reaction.

In animals other than humans, hormonal stimulus sources play a central role in the activation of maternal behavior (e.g. see Meites and Sgouris 1954:530–4). Among humans the role of such hormonal factors is less certain while external incentives and experiential factors related to mother-infant contact become most influential. The following discussion will therefore focus upon mother-infant contact as a source for charging the Maternal System.

**Infant Contact
as a Stimulus Source for
Charging the Maternal System**

The outline in Table XVIII refers to processes by which a mother's contact with the warm and tender body of her infant will tend to charge her Maternal Affectional System circuits, i.e., the Pleasure-Reward, Tranquilizing, and Parasympathetic Systems regulating the discharge of her contented, gentle, and placid behavior* as well as her visceral reactions of warmth and the flow of milk.

**TABLE XVIII
MATERNAL EMOTION AND INFANT CONTACT**

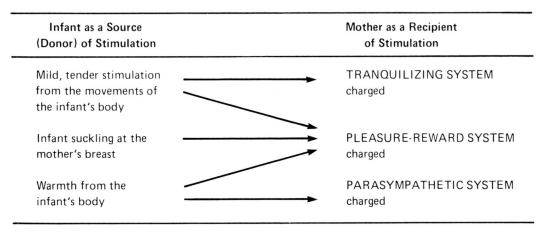

Infant as a Source (Donor) of Stimulation	Mother as a Recipient of Stimulation
Mild, tender stimulation from the movements of the infant's body	TRANQUILIZING SYSTEM charged
Infant suckling at the mother's breast	PLEASURE-REWARD SYSTEM charged
Warmth from the infant's body	PARASYMPATHETIC SYSTEM charged

* Among males "maternal" emotion would be referred to as "brotherly" or "parental" feeling. In male parents the action of testosterone which increases forcefulness would tend to counteract a capacity for these "gentle," "tender" contact reactions with an infant.

Theoretically, the *sudden interruption* of such stimulus conditions charging the Maternal System during mother-infant contact should eventuate in the reciprocally antithetical charge of the Unpleasure-Punishment, Sympathetic, and Arousal Systems (see Chapter VII) and therefore should result in the discharge of angry, hyperactive states of excitement. This conclusion accounts for the actual upset which occurs when, for example, a baby cub is suddenly removed from its mother. The maternal animal which had been placid and gentle and relaxed, suddenly becomes restless, tense, excited, and often fiercely ferocious (Altmann, 1963:243; see DeVore, 1963:315).

Charging a Mother's Maternal System During Her Own Infancy

According to the schema presented in Table XIX the discharge of a mother's maternal emotion, the discharge of her Pleasure-Reward, Tranquilizing, and Parasympathetic Systems during contact with her infant should contribute to a reciprocal activation of "maternal-like" emotion in the infant, i.e., the infant's Pleasure-Reward, Tranquilizing, and Parasympathetic Systems tend to be extrinsically activated during mother-infant contact. In this way, an infant's (upper limbic) representation of contact with a warm tender being may become permanently associated with the processes of the Tranquilizing, Pleasure-Reward, and Parasympathetic Systems. Later in life, when the female infant becomes a mother, the image of a warm, tender being (this time her own infant) will tend to reactivate the processes of her Pleasure-Reward, Tranquilizing, and Parasympathetic Systems (i.e., will tend to reactivate her maternal emotion). Conversely, a "motherless-mother" would be lacking such early emotional conditioning of positive, warm, and tranquilizing contact reactions. This conclusion is substantiated by Harlow's experimental studies (1963:275-7) which indicate that if a female monkey is deprived of a mother's contact during her infancy, she subsequently will be incapable of mothering her own infant (see Fig. IX-3).

The process of maternal affectional imprinting would be comparable to sexual imprinting in that the emotional conditioning occurring early in infancy would result in relatively irreversible effects.*

---

* Such early irreversible emotional conditioning would be in a position to provide also for human trust: the reactions of pleasure and reward, warmth, and tranquility in the presence of other human beings. A deficit in early affectional imprinting would be expected therefore to result in a disturbance in trust, i.e., a disturbance in positive pleasurable reactions to people.

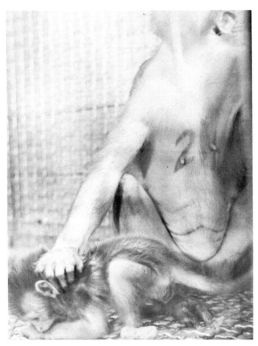

Figure IX-3. The absence of pleasurable reward-reinforcing contact response of a "motherless" mother for her infant. (Reproduced with permission, from Harlow, H.: The maternal affectional system of rhesus monkeys. In Rheingold, H., Ed.: *Maternal Behavior in Mammals*. New York: John Wiley, 1963, p. 277.)

Contrasting Non-specific Patterns of Maternal and Sexual Emotion

According to the present non-specific activation theory of emotion, both maternal and sexual emotion involve pleasure-reward activation. However, these emotions are characterized by contrasting patterns in the arousal activation of excitement (see Tables XVII and XIV). Whereas maternal emotion is involved with widespread tranquilizing effects, sexual emotion is involved with step-like increments in excitement culminating in a peak of excitement and followed by a reactive period of tranquility.

These neurophysiological concepts parallel Greenacre's (1954:19) clinical descriptions of "two types of rhythms which appear throughout life. One is the even rise and fall, the alternation of phases in a regular repetitive fashion,° subject to quite wide incidental variations, to be sure, but with a tendency to return to its essentially regular pattern. This is the rhythm of

---

° i.e., with a paucity of change characterizing non-specificity.

TABLE XIX

CHARGING "MATERNAL-LIKE" EMOTION IN THE INFANT

Maternal Emotion	The Mother as a Source of Stimulation During Mother-Infant Contact	
Discharge of mother's TRANQUILIZING SYSTEM	⟶ Diminished forcefulness of mother's responses	⟶ Outgoing stimulation of low or reduced intensity
Discharge of mother's PLEASURE-REWARD SYSTEM during infant contact	⟶ Maintenance of mother-infant contact	⟶
Discharge of mother's PARASYMPATHETIC SYSTEM	⟶ Dilatation of mother's peripheral vasculature; increased mammary gland activation	⟶ Flow of warm blood to mother's body surface; increased irradiation of warmth; increased flow of warm milk

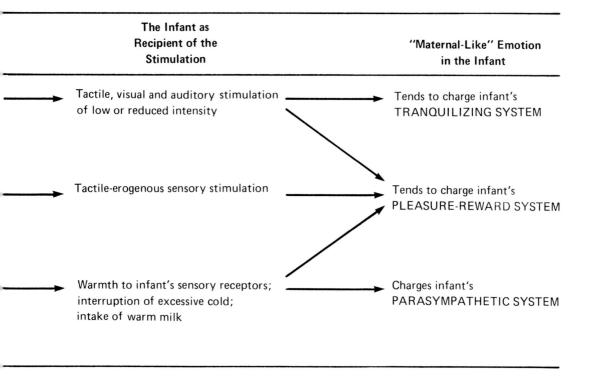

The Infant as Recipient of the Stimulation	"Maternal-Like" Emotion in the Infant
Tactile, visual and auditory stimulation of low or reduced intensity	Tends to charge infant's TRANQUILIZING SYSTEM
Tactile-erogenous sensory stimulation	Tends to charge infant's PLEASURE-REWARD SYSTEM
Warmth to infant's sensory receptors; interruption of excessive cold; intake of warm milk	Charges infant's PARASYMPATHETIC SYSTEM

day and night, or of the pulse, or of breathing, and tends to invade our voluntary activities as well. By its endless repetitiveness, and constant alternation of short-spanned change and familiarity, it is soothing and has the pleasure and assurance of the recurringly familiar. The second type of rhythm is of the climactic or orgastic kind, in which there is a gradual, usually step-like rise of mounting excitement and strain (dependent on partial frustration but with continued excitation) reaching a peak or climax of discharge with a sudden relaxation of tension and the achievement of a pitch of pleasure . . . followed by the contrasting relaxation pleasure of relief. The simple repetitive rhythm is lulling by its incessant familiarity, the orgastic type is sleep-producing through a fatigue, satiety of gratification. . . ."

In summary, sexual and maternal emotion both pertain to feelings of warmth and pleasure. However, the former involves contact reactions which eventuate in mounting often ecstatic periods of excitement, while the latter involves contact reactions which are basically empathetic: directly tranquilizing and comforting.

Chapter X

The Posterior Sensory Discriminatory Cortex

The preceding chapters have focused upon the u-h-r emotional core of the central nervous system. The remaining chapters will deal with the processes of cognition and intention as they relate to this emotional core.

An understanding of cognition and intention in terms of CNS processes requires some reference to the functions of the most highly developed region of the brain, the neocortex. Pribram (1960:1340) describes the neocortex as consisting of a posterior sensory "discriminatory" (differentiative) and an anterior "intentional" section.

Chapter X will deal with neocortical *sensory* functions.

Chapter XI will focus upon neocortical *sensory-motor* functions in relation to reward mechanisms.

Chapter XII will deal with neocortical *intentional* functions in relation to these reward mechanisms.

The Posterior Extrinsic Sensory Cortex
Neuroanatomical Considerations

"Extrinsic", as previously defined, (see Chapter II) refers to a predominance of impulses directly projected to or from the periphery of the nervous system. The extrinsic areas of the posterior sensory neocortex receive the direct thalamic projection of impulses from the peripheral sensory receptors (Rose and Woolsey, 1949:391–404). They have been referred to by a number of equivalent names as outlined in Table XX.

The location of and numerical reference to the extrinsic neocortical sensory projection areas are indicated in Table XXI and Figure X-1 (see Penfield, 1937:389–441; Krieg, 1966:871–4). These findings have been obtained by the use of implanted electrode techniques to determine points within the neocortex which react to localized stimulation of the external receptors (see Pribram, 1958:156).

TABLE XX
THE EXTRINSIC SENSORY CORTEX

Equivalent Terms*	Reference
Extrinsic sensory cortex	Rose and Woolsey, 1949:391–404
Primary sensory areas	House and Pansky, 1967:458
Primary receptive areas	Ruch, 1965:454
Sensory areas; sensory projection areas of the cortex	Hebb, 1949:124
Projective or transit sensory areas of the cortex	Konorski, 1967:84–5

*These terms will be used interchangeably.

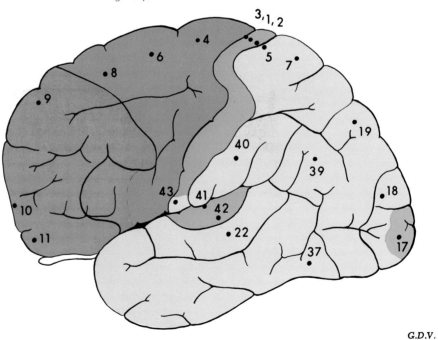

G.D.V.

Figure X-1. The extrinsic and intrinsic sectors of the neocortex: extrinsic sensory areas (dark blue), intrinsic associative sensory areas (light blue), extrinsic motor areas (green), anterior intrinsic areas including upper limbic areas (red).

TABLE XXI
EXTRINSIC AREAS OF THE SENSORY CORTEX
(According to Brodmann's Classification)

Modality	Area	Lobe
Somaesthetic and proprioceptive	1, 2, 3	Parietal
Visual	17	Occipital
Auditory	41, 42	Temporal

The Posterior Extrinsic Sensory Cortex:
Functional Properties

Sensory Reception and Discrimination

The extrinsic sensory areas of the neocortex mediate localized sensory reception. Extirpation of an extrinsic sensory area is followed by pronounced deficits or complete loss in conscious *sensation* for a given modality (Kluver, 1942:253). The organization of sensation within extrinsic sensory areas involves a *topographic projection* of impulses from the peripheral sensory receptors of a given modality. This has been demonstrated in relation to vision among monkeys by Talbot and Marshall (1941:1255–64) who recorded points of maximal electrical activity within the extrinsic visual cortex, area 17, while individual points of the retina were stimulated with a beam of light. Their studies revealed that the retina is projected like a map upon area 17, with maximal space and detail afforded to the fovea. By the use of similar techniques Woolsey, Marshall, and Bard (1942:399–439) found that the tactile areas of the body surface are represented in an orderly sequence within the extrinsic somaesthetic areas 3, 1, 2 (see Fig. IV-3). Also the individual points of the cochlea-receptor surface are projected topographically upon the extrinsic auditory cortex (Woolsey and Walzl, 1942:315–41).

Correlated with this point-to-point projection of sensory impulses is the finding that the functioning of the extrinsic sensory cortex is essential for sensory discrimination (Kluver, 1942:253). The greater the anatomical precision with which a sensory receptor surface is projected upon the extrinsic sensory cortex, the more highly developed is the associated capacity for sensory discrimination (Talbot, 1941:1255–64; Rose, 1959:402).

Non-associative Transient Traces

By definition each extrinsic sensory area of the cortex involves the direct projection of impulses from specific sensory receptors of a given modality, uninterrupted by an input from internal circuits or associative connections. Therefore the projected processes like those of the external receptors which they duplicate, involve not the association of impulses from different modalities but rather a continual series of transient traces under the control of the external environment.

The Posterior Intrinsic Sensory Cortex: Neuroanatomical Considerations

"Intrinsic" as previously defined (see Chapter II) refers to a predominance of internal circuits interrupting direct projection of impulses. The intrinsic areas of the posterior sensory cortex form internal circuits with the associational nuclei of the thalamus (Rose and Woolsey, 1949:391–404). They have been referred to by a number of equivalent terms as outlined in Table XXII.

Well-known intrinsic areas of the cerebral cortex are listed in Table XXIII and illustrated in Figure X-1 (see Krieg, W., 1966:871–4).

TABLE XXII
THE INTRINSIC SENSORY CORTEX

Equivalent Terms*	Reference
Intrinsic sensory cortex	Rose and Woolsey, 1949:391-404
Secondary sensory areas of the cortex	House and Pansky, 1967:460
The association areas of the cortex	Hebb, 1949:124
The gnostic areas	Konorski, 1967:73–75, 105

*These terms in subsequent discussions will be used interchangeably.

TABLE XXIII
INTRINSIC AREAS OF THE SENSORY CORTEX
(According to Brodmann's Classification)

Modality	Area	Lobe
Somaesthetic	5, 7, 40, 43	Parietal
Visual	18, 19, 37, 39	Occipital
Auditory	22	Temporal

Interconnections Between the Extrinsic and Intrinsic Areas of the Posterior Sensory Cortex

Two sets of findings have been reported with respect to connections between extrinsic and intrinsic sensory areas of the neocortex. According to one set of findings, there exist numerous direct connections between extrinsic and intrinsic sensory areas (route 1 in Fig. X-2) (see Crosby, 1962:459). On the other hand, Pribram presents evidence that connections between these areas take place indirectly via the associational nuclei of the thalamus (route 1a→1b in Fig. X-2) (Pribram, 1958:169).

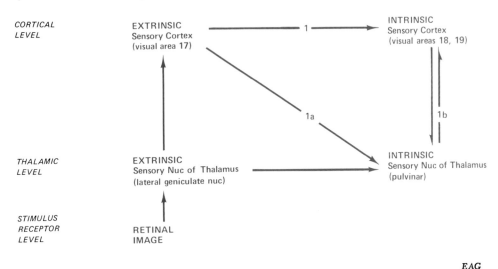

Figure X-2. Direct (1) or indirect (1a → 1b) connections between the extrinsic and intrinsic areas of the posterior discriminatory cortex.

In either case there is general agreement that impulses are relayed from the extrinsic receptive cortex to the intrinsic associative cortex:

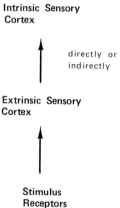

Intrinsic Sensory
Cortex

directly or
indirectly

Extrinsic Sensory
Cortex

Stimulus
Receptors

Neuroanatomical Connections, a Symbolic Presentation

Konorski (1967:64–5) writes that these connections from the receptors of the body surface to the extrinsic (projective) areas and from there to the intrinsic (gnostic) areas form different but connected "levels" of organization within each ascending sensory system for a given modality. Only at the top intrinsic level are branching connections formed between modality systems.

These conclusions may be outlined succinctly in terms of the following symbols derived from Hebb (1949:85–90) and Konorski (1967:65):

Let

a, b, c = *external stimulus* conditions
a′, b′, c′ = *extrinsic* projective sensory representations respectively pertaining to stimulus conditions a, b, c
a″,b″,c″ = *intrinsic* associative, gnostic, representations respectively pertaining to stimulus conditions a, b, c

Konorski's description of the interrelation between various levels of sensory organization according to which the peripheral reception of external stimuli innervates extrinsic (projective) images that in turn innervate intrinsic (gnostic) representations may be symbolically represented as follows:

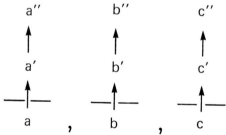

The Posterior Intrinsic Sensory Cortex:
Functional Properties

Pooling of Sensory Contributions

Although the input into an extrinsic sensory area of the thalamus or cortex involves afferent impulses of only a single sensory modality, the input into an intrinsic associational area often derives from a number of different modality areas. Intrinsic somaesthetic areas 5 and 7, for example, receive fibres from the visual and auditory cortex (see Crosby, 1962:449).

The importance of pooling in the formation of associative representations within the intrinsic sensory cortex becomes evident in the light of clinical pathology. Gesell and Amatruda (1947:258) point out: "The senses were meant to function in synaesthesia, two or more modalities blending. Even the primary tactual sense does not normally function in pure form. Tactual perceptions are also visual-tactual perceptions for the normal mind. If this close reciprocal interacting relationship between vision and touch is not recognized, it is impossible to appreciate the gravity of the handicap under which the blind and near-blind infant labors." Hebb (1949:79–106) concludes that visual perception is determined by visual and proprioceptive pooling: he points out how proprioceptive feedback from eye movements may contribute to visual perceptual integration. Likewise, Konorski (1967:230–2) notes that intrinsic (gnostic) area pooling of contributions from auditory, visual, and proprioceptive sensory modalities are essential for the formation of verbal representations.

Formation of Memory Trace Engrams

The actual nature of traces is still unknown. However, new lines of research are developing in the fields of neurophysiology and molecular chemistry to probe into the nature of processes which account for memory. Research (see Hydén, 1970:101–18) suggests that memory traces are a function of the modification of cortical neuronal cells involving chemical constituents within the cells or synaptic arrangement of numerous terminal knobs. In either case there is general agreement that memory traces involve the formation of new patterns of cell firing.

Opinions have differed as to whether trace engrams are localized within specific areas of the cortex or whether they are a general function of activities within the total cortex. Lashley (1929) favored the concept that the cortex has a "mass action" effect in that most cortical lesions interfere equally with learning. More recent studies such as those involving the sectioning of the corpus collosum (Sperry, 1958:418) suggest that a single stimulus may provide for more than one trace and that multiple storage of individual memory traces is responsible for the mass action of the cortex in learning. The studies of Bykov in Pavlov's laboratory and more recent studies of Myers and Sperry have convinced Sperry (ibid:418) that "one is not misled after all in continuing to search for specific functions in the various centers and connecting fibre systems of the brain. . . ." e.g. with respect to memory (See Ruch, 1965:489).

Neuroanatomically, the posterior intrinsic sensory cortex is in an optimal position to serve the formation of long-lasting sensory memory traces:

1. It is a sensory cortex whose input involves relay of impulses from numerous extrinsic projection sensory areas. Its processes therefore are in a position to provide for the pooled sensory aspects of memory.

2. The reverberatory properties of the intrinsic° areas provide a most likely source for repetitive activation of those chemical or physical processes that are essential for the establishment of long-lasting memory traces (John, 1967:28–40).

The intrinsic sensory cortex thus is in a better position to provide for prolonged sensory memory traces than is the extrinsic sensory cortex whose functions involve principally the formation of transient traces.

Sperry's concept of multiple representation of memory traces suggests that other areas of the cortex also contribute to memory. The possible part played by the prefrontal limbic cortex in the formation and storage of "emotional" memories will be considered in Chapter XII.

Association of Sensory Representations with One Another

The associative connections of the intrinsic sensory cortex provide a possible basis for not only (1) the formation of memory traces or representations via the pooling of contributions from many sensory modalities but also (2) the interrelation of such representations (Konorski, 1967:189).

The association between sensory representations, S→S learning, has been substantiated by behavioral studies (see Kimble, 1961:235–7). Neurophysiological techniques also have been used to demonstrate such associations. For example, Durup and Fessard (1935:1–32; see also Konorski, 1967:189) have shown that if a sound and a visual stimulus are repeatedly paired, eventually the sound by itself may elicit within the visual cortex EEG changes which originally were elicited only by the visual stimulus.

The establishment of associational connections between different intrinsic trace sensory representations may be symbolically indicated as follows:

° "Intrinsic" has been defined in terms of the predominance of reverberating circuits interrupting direct projection (see Chapter II).

(1) Let

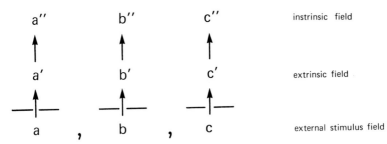

(2) and let stimulus, a, be paired in sequence with stimulus b and c so that representation of, a, is paired with representation of b and with representation of c:

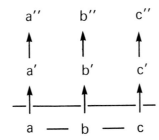

(3) then these procedures provide a basis for associative connections between intrinsic sensory trace representations a″, b″ and c″[*]:

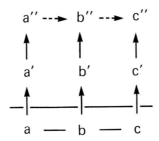

(4) so that on future occasions:

$$a'' \longrightarrow b'' \longrightarrow c''$$

This formulation pertaining to the association of intrinsic sensory representations is equivalent to the concept of the temporal association of thoughts or ideas.

[*] It will be recalled there is little opportunity for formation of associations at the extrinsic field level and association occurs primarily at the intrinsic field level.

Learning

Evidence has been presented indicating that the posterior intrinsic sensory cortex serves (1) the formation of intrinsic (gnostic) memory traces and (2) the association between such intrinsic traces. These processes provide the essentials of cognitive learning (Konorski, 1967:86–90; see also Grossman, 1967:815–46, 879–80).

Summary

The *extrinsic* posterior sensory cortex provides for discriminatory sensation: transient, topographical reception of impulses projected from sensory receptors of a given modality. The *intrinsic* posterior sensory cortex provides for the formation of long-lasting memory traces and for the associative interrelation of these traces, processes which are important for cognitive learning.

Conjoint Functions of the Extrinsic and Intrinsic Posterior Sensory Cortices

Perception

Stimulus perception may be analyzed in terms of (1) external stimuli, (2) accompanying sensations, and (3) their associative images and thoughts or "meaning." These factors have already been discussed as functions of stimuli a, b, c, their corresponding extrinsic or projective sensory processes a', b', c', and their intrinsic associative or gnostic processes a", b", c". Perception of a, b, c, may be represented by the formulae:

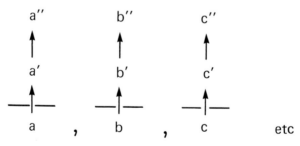

Perceptual Expectation

A definition of expectation in terms of neurophysiological constructs may be derived as follows:

(1) Let a sequence of stimuli a, b, c, presented to the subject be indicated symbolically by a − b − c.

(2) Let this sequence be accompanied by a sequential perception of the stimuli:

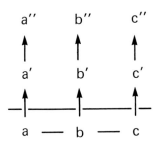

then (3) according to Konorski's formulation pertaining to the association of intrinsic or "gnostic" representations, the following processes of association may take place:

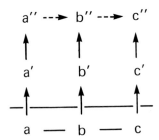

and

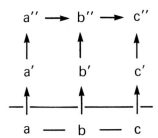

so that

In this way, the intrinsic representations b″ and c″ may be innervated without the current presentation of stimuli b and c, and without the innervation of the corresponding extrinsic sensory processes b′ and c′; b″ and c″ are innervated without direct innervation of perceptions:

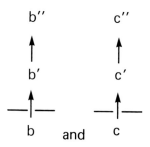

These statements rephrase Konorski's hypothesis (1967:170) that an intrinsic (gnostic) representation, c″, may be activated in either of two ways: "either from the periphery through afferent pathways":

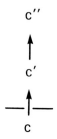

"or. . . . through associative pathways":

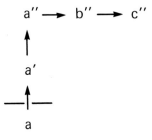

It becomes evident that reintroduction of, a, the stimulus which occurred early in the sequence, a–b–c, now elicits the representation of, c, the stimulus which occurred later in that sequence. This formulation coincides with the everyday definition of expectation illustrated by the following example: If an individual has been exposed to the stimulus sequence: axe hits tree – tree is severed – tree falls, subsequent observation of the axe hitting the tree (the reintroduction of the stimulus which occurred early in the original sequence) elicits an "expectation" of the tree falling (elicits a representation of the stimulus which occurred later in the same sequence). This definition of perceptual expectation may be formulated scientifically in terms of the following three operational procedures:

(1) presentation of a stimulus sequence:

$$a - b - c$$

(2) verbal notation of perceptual awareness of each stimulus presented in sequence:

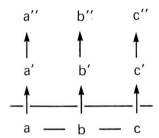

(3) verbal notation as to whether the reintroduction of the stimulus, a, now elicits the representation or thought of the stimulus, c, according to the prediction:

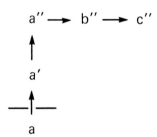

In summary, perceptual expectation is defined as a process whereby the presentation of a stimulus which occurred early in a sequence elicits the representation of a stimulus which occurred later in the sequence.

This formulation is basically equivalent to that which Beritashvili (1969: 653–4) derived from his physio-psychological studies. It is further elaborated in Appendix II in relation to spatial perceptual expectations and the Gestalt phenomenon of closure.[*]

For S-R psychologists who conceive of representations as consisting not of central nervous system reactions, but as peripheral "partial responses," the above definition of expectation may be expressed in terms

---

[*] See also Appendix III for a consideration of expectations as a function of verbal stimuli.

of such partial responses, r_a, r_b, r_c (see Kimble, 1961:234) as follows:

$$r_a \longrightarrow r_b \longrightarrow r_c$$
$$\uparrow$$
$$S_a$$

rather than as

$$a'' \longrightarrow b'' \longrightarrow c''$$
$$\uparrow$$
$$a'$$
$$\uparrow$$
$$a$$

They would refer to the innervation of r_c rather than of c'' as occurring prior to the appearance of the actual event, c.

Expectation Confirmed by Perception

Expectation of, c, confirmed by perception of, c, may be schematically noted as follows:

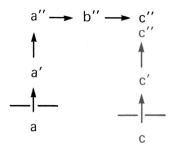

When perception of, c, confirms expectation of, c, (1) c'' is first facilitated intrinsically or centrally by expectation:

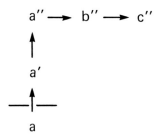

and (2) then is facilitated extrinsically or sensorily by perception:

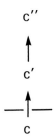

This description reflects Hebb's conclusions (1949:87fn): "'Expectancy' implies that. . . . central facilitation . . . precedes the sensory. . . ."

Expectation Unconfirmed by Perception

Expectation of, c, unconfirmed by perception may be schematically noted as follows:

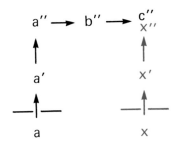

In terms of the preceding example, the expectation of observing the tree falling ($\rightarrow$ c") is unconfirmed when instead there occurs a percep-

tion of the tree floating through the air 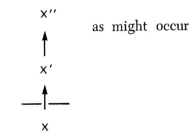 as might occur

during a theatrical performance of a children's fairy tale.

According to Konorski (1967:182), mutual antagonism between two concomitantly activated but discrepant intrinsic (gnostic) representations eventuates in the inhibition of the less stable representation. He also proposes that actual perception usually suppresses all images antagonistic to it. Thus a discrepancy between perception and expectation should eventuate in the predominance of the perceptual image.

Neocortical Perceptual-Motor Functions

Perceptual-motor functions are organized within the posterior sensory and the central motor areas of the cerebral cortex (see Fig. X-1).

Symbolic Presentation of Perceptual-Motor Processes

The use of the symbols

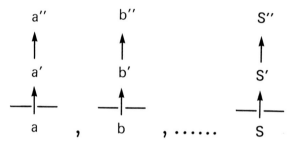

to denote sensory perception suggests the use of an equivalent set of symbols

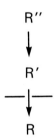

to denote the pyramidal motor engrams involved with the control of specific response, R:

> R' = an extrinsic neocortical, pyramidal motor engram governing response, R, e.g., a motor engram within areas 4 or 6 (see Fig. X-1).

where "extrinsic" pertains to predominance of direct connections with the peripheral musculature, i.e., without interruption from internal circuits.

> R'' = an intrinsic associative neocortical engram pertaining to response, R, e.g. a proprioceptive engram within areas 5 or 7;

where "intrinsic" pertains to the predominance of internal circuits interrupting direct connections with the peripheral musculature.

Posterior intrinsic sensory areas 5 and 7 are involved with motor as well as proprioceptive, somaesthetic sensory representation (Crosby, 1962:

449–50). These areas with their widespread associational connections therefore provide one possible locus for perceptual-motor associations:

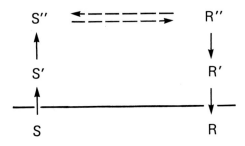

This formulation incorporates Konorski's conclusion that association takes place primarily at intrinsic levels.*

Chapter XI will focus upon the question as to how these specific neocortical perceptual-motor processes may be affected by u-h-r non-specific reinforcement mechanisms.

---

* The extrinsic sensory areas do mediate some sensory-motor reflexes. However, these are limited to localized automatic reactions which serve sensory orientation: eye movements are elicited from the visual extrinsic sensory areas, ear movements from the auditory extrinsic areas, etc. (Walker, 1940:353–7; Bechterew, 1911:1859–64). Konorski (1967:17) refers to these as target reflexes which do not involve complex conditional associational learning.

Chapter XI

The Arousal, Reward, and
Punishment of Behavior

Two types of behavioral reinforcement have been shown to be intimately associated with processes of the u-h-r systems (see Tables VIII and IV): (1) arousal reinforcement of the *magnitude,* intensity, or forcefulness of response; (2) reward reinforcement of the *maintenance* or continuance and repetition of response.

U-H-R Arousal System Reinforcement
of the Magnitude of Response

Lindsley's studies have drawn attention to the synergistic interaction of the specific perceptual-motor and the ascending non-specific activating systems (see Chapter II). Low levels of non-specific activation result in diminished arousal of sensory perception and motor behavior; conversely, high levels of non-specific activation result in elevated arousal. The diagram in Figure XI–1 schematically depicts the synergistic interaction of the specific perceptual-motor and non-specific activating systems as a basis for non-specific reinforcement of the magnitude (intensity, forcefulness) of perceptual-motor response. Extrinsic sensory and motor engrams, S′ and R′, are each shown to be (a) specifically innervated and (b) non-specifically activated.

The significance of moment-to-moment changes in the level of ascending phasic non-specific activation affecting specifically innervated perceptual-motor engrams may be illustrated by the following example:

Let $\quad$ S $\ =$ a visual stimulus pattern pertaining to an object placed a short distance below the subject's hand

$\qquad$ S′ $=$ the corresponding extrinsic visual photographic image

and let

$\qquad$ R $=$ the motor response of moving the hand downward upon the object

$\qquad$ R′ $=$ the corresponding extrinsic motor engrams governing response, R

Then, if the motor engram, R′, for moving the hand downward is specific-

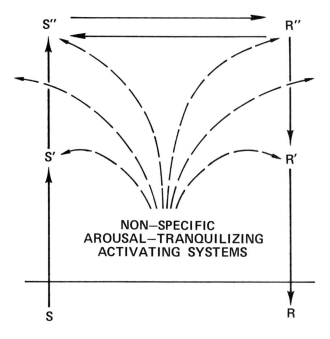

NON—SPECIFIC
AROUSAL—TRANQUILIZING
ACTIVATING SYSTEMS

EAG

Figure XI-1. Non-specific arousal activation *reinforcing the intensity* of extrinsic sensory motor processes (or non-specific tranquilizing activation inhibiting the intensity of extrinsic sensory motor processes).

ally innervated and is synergistically reinforced by Tranquilizing System discharge at low levels of phasic non-specific activation, the intensity or magnitude of the response should be low, the contact gentle. If this same sequence is reinforced by higher levels of Arousal System phasic non-specific activation, the response becomes forceful, the contact heavy. Finally, with reinforcement at highest levels of non-specific activation, the response becomes still more forceful so that the contact becomes converted into a powerful blow. In these examples, the specific response remains a constant, while the phasic non-specific arousal activation of its forcefulness, aggressiveness, or intensity varies.[*]

U-H-R Reward System Reinforcement
of the Maintenance of Response

The neurophysiological studies of Olds and of Heath demonstrate that the discharge of the non-specific Pleasure-Reward System circuits (see Chapters I–III) contributes to the reinforcement of the contin-

[*] See Appendix I for a comparison with Breuer and Freud's concepts of "intracerebral tonic excitation."

uation and repetition of on-going specific sensory-motor response. Olds (1964:26–7) writes: "A number of differences have been observed between the positive reinforcement produced by hypothalamic stimulation and that produced by rhinencephalic* stimulation . . . Animals pressed a lever 10,000 times an hour to stimulate the lateral hypothalamus but only about 500 times an hour under the same conditions to stimulate the septal or amygdaloid areas both of which are subdivisions of the rhinencephalon. The animals' 'appetites' for lateral hypothalamic stimulation often seemed relatively insatiable, whereas definite satiation was usually reached in experiments with rhinencephalic stimulation. Animals stimulated themselves several thousand times in the septal areas and then stopped for the day; animals stimulated themselves hour after hour in the lateral hypothalamus, maintaining a rate of several thousand responses per hour and stopping only when a state of physical exhaustion appeared." Such experimental data clearly demonstrate u-h-r Reward System reinforcement of the maintenance and repetition of specific on-going perceptual-motor response sequences.

The question immediately arises as to how Reward System discharge could reinforce on-going behavior. A non-specific activation theory of reward offers a possible explanation of this phenomenon. This theory proposes that reward and pleasure consist of different aspects of the same process. Pleasure would consist of the effects of certain patterns of ascending phasic non-specific activation upon perceptual consciousness; reward, the effects of these patterns of non-specific activation upon the maintenance of on-going sensory-motor behavior.

The diagram in Figure XI–2 illustrates this concept. It refers to u-h-r contributions to unique patterns of non-specific activation reinforcing the reverberation of the associative $S'' \rightleftharpoons R''$ circuits, a neurophysiological basis for the maintenance of the on-going specific sensory-motor activity.

U-H-R Punishment System Negative Effects
upon the Maintenance of Response

Olds' (1964:30–3) and Lilly's (1958:705–20) experimental findings demonstrate that the discharge of the Punishment System circuits contributes to the disruption of on-going response. Olds notes (ibid:32) that while purely positive reinforcement of behavior is produced by stimulation of the lateral hypothalamic tube, purely negative effects are produced by stimulation of the periventricular system of fibres.

---

* i.e., the upper limbic areas

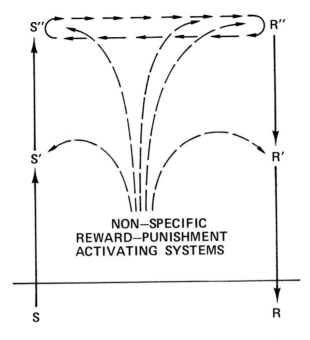

EAG

Figure XI-2. Non-specific reward activation is shown *reinforcing* the reverberation of the intrinsic S″ ⇌ R″ circuit processes and the maintenance of corresponding sensory-motor behavior. Similarly, non-specific punishment activation may disrupt the maintenance of the S″ ⇌ R″ circuit processes and the maintenance of the corresponding sensory-motor behavior.

A non-specific activation theory of unpleasure and punishment proposes that both unpleasure and punishment involve certain patterns of ascending phasic non-specific activation. Unpleasure would involve effects upon perception; punishment, the disruptive effects upon the maintenance of on-going sensory-motor processes. The diagram in Figure XI–2 suggests a mechanism by which central reverberating associative processes maintaining a conditional sensory-motor reaction may be inhibited or disrupted by certain discordant rhythmic patterns of ascending non-specific activation.

Charging the Non-specific
U-H-R Reward-Punishment System Circuits

If pleasure and reward consist of different aspects of the same process, then the Reward System is the Pleasure System, and conditions charging the one are those which charge the other. Similarly, the conditions which

TABLE XXIV
PRIMARY CONDITIONS CHARGING THE PUNISHMENT SYSTEM

1. Pain receptor stimulation and certain specialized receptor (e.g., gustatory) stimulation (via thalamic reticulum)

2. Excessive muscular tension associated with interruptions of the discharge of innervated response (probably via reticular formation)

3. Metabolic, physical, endocrine stimulation (via hypothalamic internal sensory receptors, e.g., during food or water deprivation)

4. Emotional conditioning (via upper limbic areas)

5. Excess arousal stimulation (via reticular formation)

6. Deficiency of arousal stimulation (via reticular formation)

7. Interruption of conditions charging the Reward System (e.g., via reticular formation, hypothalamus, and upper limbic areas)

TABLE XXV
PRIMARY CONDITIONS CHARGING THE REWARD SYSTEM

1. Erotogenic receptor stimulation and other specialized receptor (e.g., gustatory) stimulation (presumably via thalamic reticulum)

2. Reduction of excessive muscular tension associated with the release or discharge of innervated response (probably via reticular formation)

3. Metabolic, physical, endocrine stimulation (via hypothalamic internal sensory receptors, e.g., during food or water intake)

4. Emotional conditioning[*] (via upper limbic areas)

5. A modicum of arousal stimulation[†] (via reticular formation)

6. A modicum of tranquilizing stimulation[‡] (via reticular formation)

7. Interruption of conditions charging the Punishment System[§] (via reticular formation, hypothalamus, and upper limbic areas)

[*]i.e., secondary reward learning: the conditioning of stimuli to elicit reward mechanisms

[†]This would include a modicum of stimulus specificity, stimulus change, i.e., novelty as a source for charging the Reward System. This concept offers a non-animistic explanation of the "drive" for novelty or for exploration.

[‡]This would include a modicum of stimulus non-specificity, i.e., stimulus constancy as a source for charging the Reward System, a concept which offers an explanation for the "drive" for the "familiar."

[§]Reward effects which derive from the interruption of conditions charging the Punishment System have been referred to by behavioral therapists as "escape-reinforcement" or "negative-reinforcement" (Reese, 1966:20). Numerous experimental studies (Lindsley, 1957:1290; Azrin, 1962:781; Hefferline, 1959:1338) have demonstrated the effectiveness of this source of reward reinforcement.

charge the Punishment System must be those which charge its counterpart, the Unpleasure System. Tables XXIV and XXV list these conditions.

U-H-R Reward and Punishment System
Effects upon the Maintenance of Contact Response

Non-specific reward reinforcement of any on-going sensory-motor contact response should result in the maintenance of that response. For example, if a visual, olfactory, or auditory contact response is accompanied by reward non-specific activation, then this contact would tend to be maintained. Reward reinforcement of such a contact response therefore would provide for what is psychologically referred to as attraction, specific attention, acceptance, or positive orientation. Conversely, non-specific punishment disruption of any on-going sensory-motor contact would provide for change of that contact response, referred to psychologically as reactions of avoidance, rejection, or repulsion.

Physiological experimental studies confirm the conclusions that stimulation of the u-h-r Reward System results in the prolongation of sensory-motor contacts. Hernandez-Péon (1964:214) refers to these prolongation effects when upper limbic areas are stimulated: "A state of prolonged attention (magnetic attention) to otherwise unattractive objects (a pencil, for example) has been obtained in animals with a poorly developed cortex, such as the cat, by localized cholinergic stimulation of the septal region." And Grastyan (1959:119) writes of prolongation of contact responses when the hypothalamus and reticular formation are stimulated: "Some years ago, when studying the effect of electrical stimulation of the hypothalamus and the reticular formation . . . we were surprised to see that stimulation of certain points resulted in a phenomenon differing markedly from the usual picture . . . If . . . a moving object were brought into the visual field of the cat during stimulation, the animal was attracted by it and *riveted* to it as if it had been a magnet." The author labels such a reaction a "sensory fixation reaction."

The reverse effect, contact-response disruption eventuating in avoidance or escape, has been referred to by Lilly (1958:707, Table I) and by Olds (1964:49, 32 including Fig. 6). Olds' emphasis upon the repelling, avoidance or escape effects accompanying stimulation of the Punishment System during sensory-motor contact is reflected by his designation of this system as "the Substrate of Escape."

When activated during sensory-motor contacts, the Reward System is a positive system which reinforces contact (a source for attraction) and the Punishment is a negative system which elicits disruption of contact (a source for repulsion). Anokhin (see Diamond, 1963:213) emphasizes the importance in the behavioral repertoire of animals of "the positive-accepting response" and "the negative-rejecting response." Lilly (1958: 707) points out that the positive system elicits stimulus contact perpetuation, the negative system elicits stimulus contact termination.

Additionally when (1) a visual, olfactory, or auditory *contact response* (2) is coupled with *forward locomotion,* and then (3) reinforced by *reward activation,* the result is stimulus approach. If it is disrupted by punishment activation, the result is cessation or disruption of approach, that is, withdrawal or avoidance. Olds (1964:49) refers to these approach and avoidance aspects of the reward and punishment systems and notes that hypothalamic and paleocortical mechanisms control the basic directions of behavior: "toward some things and away from others."

In summary, it is proposed that the discharge of the non-specific Reward System reinforces the *maintenance of* (1) sensory-motor response, (2) sensory-motor contact response, a basis for stimulus attraction, and (3) sensory-motor visual contact response during locomotion, a basis for stimulus approach.

Conversely, the discharge of the non-specific Punishment System results in the *disruption of* (1) sensory-motor response, (2) sensory-motor contact response, a basis for stimulus aversion or avoidance, and (3) sensory-motor visual contact response during locomotion, a basis for escape.[*]

Insofar as the Reward and Punishment Systems determine which responses will be continued or discontinued, these systems regulate the *selection* of behavior. Insofar as these same systems determine which *approach* responses are continued or discontinued, they determine the *direction* of behavior. Reward-Punishment System regulation of selection and direction of behavior supplements Arousal System regulation of the forcefulness of behavior. Together the effects of these two activating systems account for what Young (1961:24) refers to as the two most important aspects of motivation: those pertaining to energy and direction. He refers to the concept of motivation as "the process of arousing action (and) sustaining the activity . . . ," exactly those processes which are served by the Arousal-Tranquilizing and the Reward-Punishment non-specific activating systems.

The paramecium's *protoplasm* reacting diffusely to chemical, thermal, and tactile stimulation within the external environment regulates the magnitude and selection-direction of its contact responses (see Diamond, 1963:68–9). Equivalently, the vertebrate's *Arousal-Tranquilizing* and

---

[*] These formulations apply to conditionally not to unconditionally determined behavior.

Reward-Punishment non-specific activating systems, reacting to external and internal stimulus conditions, regulate the magnitude and selection-direction of the vertebrate's contact reactions with the environment. These non-specific activating systems therefore serve functions which truly form the core of plastic, adaptive behavior.

Chapter XII

Interaction of the Processes of the Posterior "Discriminatory" Cortex with Those of the Anterior "Intentional" Cortex

The Anterior Intrinsic Cortex

Pribram (1960:1340) has emphasized the contrasting functions of the posterior "discriminatory" and anterior "intentional" cortices. The latter consists of prefrontal and orbito-temporal areas which form a neocortical extension of the upper limbic system (Nauta, 1964:405; also see Fig. X–1). Pribram's reference to the anterior areas as "intentional" is in keeping with experimental findings that they are closely associated with the u-h-r systems whose stimulation activates reactions of reward and punishment.

Symbolic Reference to Representations Within the Anterior Intrinsic Upper Limbic Cortex

Whereas representations within the posterior extrinsic sensory cortex have been denoted by the symbols a′, b′, c′ . . . and those of the posterior intrinsic sensory cortex by a″, b″, c″ . . . the corresponding representations within the intentional anterior intrinsic upper limbic cortex will be denoted by a‴, b‴, c‴.

The thalamic input of the anterior intrinsic upper limbic cortex, the innervation of a‴, b‴, c‴, has been previously summarized in Figure II–10. The efferent output of the anterior intrinsic cortex via the nonspecific Pleasure-Reward, Unpleasure-Punishment, and the Arousal and Tranquilizing Systems may be denoted symbolically as in Figure XII–1. The diagrams refer to the anatomical pathways outlined in Figures II–7, II–8, and II–9.

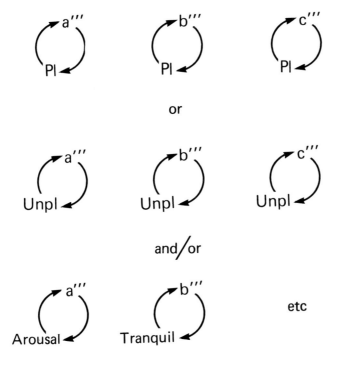

or

and/or

etc

EAG

Figure XII-1. The emotional output of the anterior-intrinsic upper limbic cortex: a symbolic presentation.

Together, the thalamic input and the Pleasure-Reward System output of this area may be referred to in the following manner:

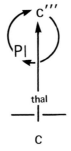

Symbolic Presentation of the Simultaneous Innervation of the Posterior Discriminatory and Anterior Intentional Cortices

The simultaneous innervation of (1) a perception within the posterior "discriminatory" cortex and (2) a Pleasure-Reward System representation within the anterior upper limbic "intentional" cortex may be referred to in the following manner:

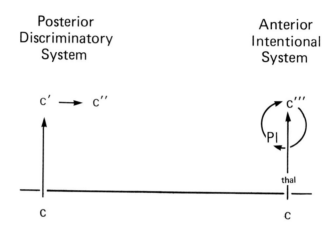

where the symbols c' and c'' refer respectively to extrinsic and intrinsic sensory representations, and c''' refers to a corresponding representation within the Pleasure-Reward System circuits. This form lends itself to a symbolic presentation of the non-specific irradiation of impulses distributed throughout the total cerebral cortex. The effects of Pleasure-Reward System activation upon posterior sensory perception therefore may be indicated as follows:

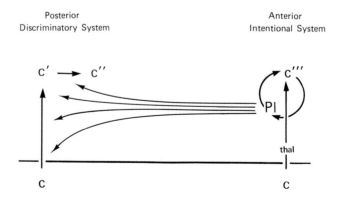

The same schematic form lends itself to a depiction of reverberatory processes that mediate the continued activation of Pleasure-Reward System representations even after termination of the initiating stimulus, c:

Posterior
Discriminatory System

Anterior
Intentional System

The interaction of a specifically innervated perceptual expectation with the non-specific processes of the Pleasure-Reward System would then be indicated as follows:

Posterior
Discriminatory System

Anterior
Intentional System

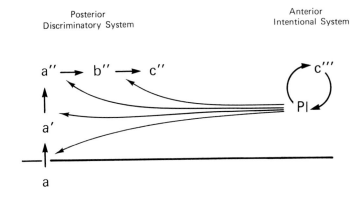

Connections Between
the Posterior Sensory
and the Anterior Intentional Cortices

Connections between the posterior sensory (occipito-parieto-temporal) and the anterior upper limbic intentional (frontal-orbito-insular-temporal) cortices involve some of the most prominent association fibres of the cerebrum. Among these are the following bundles (Kappers, 1936:1472–4): (1) the superior longitudinal fasciculus, (2) the inferior longitudinal fasciculus, (3) the superior occipito-frontal fasciculus, and (4) the inferior occipito-frontal fasciculus. The extensive distribution of these fibres is best demonstrated diagrammatically by the following illustrations from House and Pansky (1967:24):

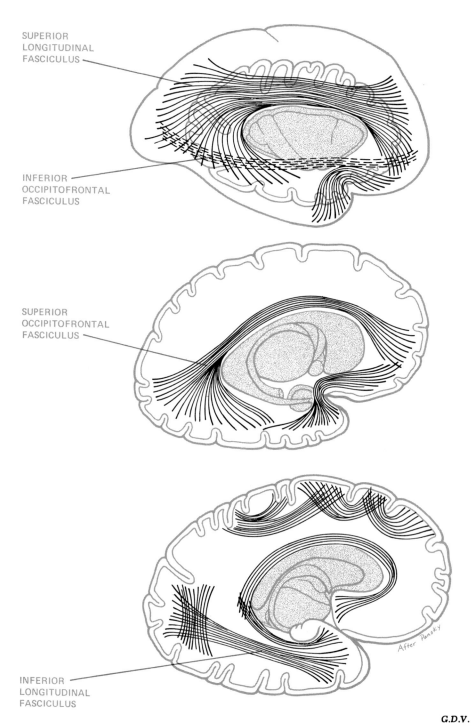

SUPERIOR
LONGITUDINAL
FASCICULUS

INFERIOR
OCCIPITOFRONTAL
FASCICULUS

SUPERIOR
OCCIPITOFRONTAL
FASCICULUS

INFERIOR
LONGITUDINAL
FASCICULUS

G.D.V.

Figure XII-2. Long and short association bundles of the cerebral cortex. (Redrawn with permission, from House, E., and Pansky, B.: *A Functional Approach to Neuroanatomy*, 2nd ed. New York: McGraw-Hill, 1967, p. 24.)

Thus, a basis for connections exists not only between the representations of the extrinsic and intrinsic posterior sensory cortices

$$c \longrightarrow c' \longrightarrow c''$$

but also between those of the posterior sensory and anterior limbic intentional cortices (Van Hoesen, 1972:1471–3):

$$\left(c' \longrightarrow c'' \right) \longrightarrow c'''$$

Furthermore, according to the laws of conditioning, reinforcement of connections tends to occur between simultaneously innervated representations.* Therefore, when c', c'', $c''' \rightarrow$ Pl are simultaneously innervated, their connections will tend to be reinforced:

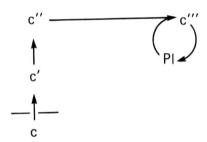

The Concept of Matching Representations
Within the Perceptual and Pleasure Systems

When momentary perception matches a representation activated within the Pleasure (Reward) System:

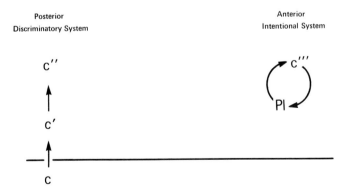

---

* It is possible that $c'' \rightarrow c'''$ may not involve the establishment of *connections* between traces but rather the establishment of *traces* at connected neural points i.e. during concomitant innervation of these connected neural points. See footnote p 99.

the innervation of perception

$$\begin{array}{c} c'' \\ \uparrow \\ c' \\ \uparrow \\ -|- \\ c \end{array}$$

should elevate the charge of the

Pleasure (Reward) System circuit via the pathways shown:

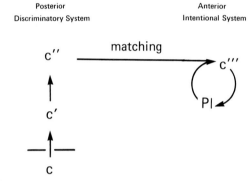

which may be also expressed as:

$$c \longrightarrow c' \longrightarrow c'' \longrightarrow c''' \longrightarrow PI$$

or,

In the above schematic presentation, the connections $c \to c' \to c'' \to c'''$ are understood to have been established in the past. The reintroduction of stimulus c, then, is in a position to reactivate these connections and the Pleasure System circuit

On the other hand, when momentary perception does not match a representation activated within the Pleasure System:

$$x'' \xrightarrow{\text{not matching}} \left(\begin{array}{c} c''' \\ PI \end{array} \right)$$

$$\begin{array}{c} x'' \\ \uparrow \\ x' \\ \uparrow \\ ---\uparrow--- \\ x \end{array}$$

then perception does not charge the Pleasure System circuit

$$x \rightarrow x' \rightarrow x'' \xrightarrow{\text{not matching}} (c'' \rightarrow PI)$$

Theoretically, when perception ($c \rightarrow c' \rightarrow c''$) matching a Pleasure System representation is replaced by perception ($x \rightarrow x' \rightarrow x''$) not matching the Pleasure System representation, perceptual reinforcement of the Pleasure System charge is interrupted or reduced. This reduction contributes to a reciprocally antithetical increment in the charge of the Unpleasure System (see Chapter VII). These reactions are indicated by the following formula:

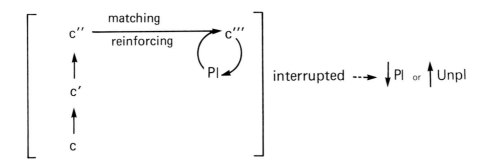

The Concept of Matching Perceptual Expectation and Pleasure System Representations

A sensory perceptual expectation has been defined as a process whereby a stimulus, a, which occurred early in a sequence, a–b–c, may elicit a sensory representation of stimulus, c, which occurred later in the sequence:

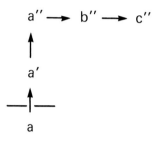

Innervation of a perceptual expectation occurring simultaneously with the activation of a corresponding representation within the Pleasure System would then be indicated as follows:

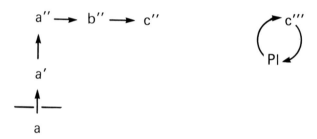

According to the hypothesis proposed in the preceding section, the association fibres within the cerebral cortex can provide for connections between a posterior intrinsic representation, c″, and its corresponding anterior intrinsic upper limbic representation, c‴. This connection would make possible an interaction not only of perception but also of perceptual expectation with representations activated within the Pleasure System:

It becomes evident that in this case perceptual expectation:

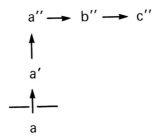

will reinforce the charge of the Pleasure System circuit via the pathways shown below:

$$a \longrightarrow a' \longrightarrow a'' \longrightarrow b'' \longrightarrow c'' \xrightarrow[\text{reinforcing}]{\text{matching}} c''' \, {}^{*}$$

or

$$\left[\begin{array}{c} a'' \longrightarrow b'' \longrightarrow c'' \xrightarrow{\text{matching}} c''' \\ \uparrow \\ a' \\ \uparrow \\ a \end{array}\right] \longrightarrow \uparrow Pl$$

If expectation matching a representation activated within the Pleasure System elevates Pleasure System charge, then interruption of this process should reduce this charge and contribute to reciprocally antithetical increments in the charge of the Unpleasure System. That is:

$$\left[\begin{array}{c} a'' \longrightarrow b'' \longrightarrow c'' \xrightarrow{\text{matching}} c''' \\ \uparrow \\ a' \\ \uparrow \\ a \end{array}\right] \text{interrupted} \longrightarrow \downarrow Pl \text{ or } \uparrow Unpl$$

* Matching of posterior cortical perceptual expectation with anterior limbic cortical representations is described more fully in Appendix V.

The following postulates summarize these conclusions pertaining to perception or perceptual expectation matching Pleasure (Reward) System representations:

Postulate I

Perception or perceptual expectation matching an activated Pleasure System representation increases the charge of the Pleasure System.

Postulate II

Interruption of perception or perceptual expectation matching an activated Pleasure System representation reduces the charge of the Pleasure System.*

Matching Perceptual Expectation with Pleasure System Representations: Sensory-Motor Effects

Matching of perceptual expectation ($\rightarrow c''$) with representations within

the Pleasure-Reward System $\left(\overset{\nearrow c'''}{\underset{Pl \nwarrow}{}} \right)$ should eventuate not only in in-

creased perceptual awareness of pleasure, but also in heightened reward reinforcement of sensory-motor behavior.†

The diagram in Figure XII–3 summarizes these processes.

The formulation is essentially the same as that derived within the preceding section. Additionally the diagram indicates that a sensory-motor response R_s takes place when motor engram R'' is activated and discharges in the presence of stimulus, s. The notation R_s — a, indicates that the sensory-motor response, R_s, is a source for stimulus, a, which in turn elicits expectation

$$a \longrightarrow a' \longrightarrow a'' \longrightarrow b'' \longrightarrow c'' \xrightarrow{\text{matching}} \overset{\nearrow c'''}{\underset{Pl \nwarrow}{}}$$

---

* See Appendix IV for a consideration of a similar set of postulates pertaining to the Unpleasure System.

† See Chapter XI.

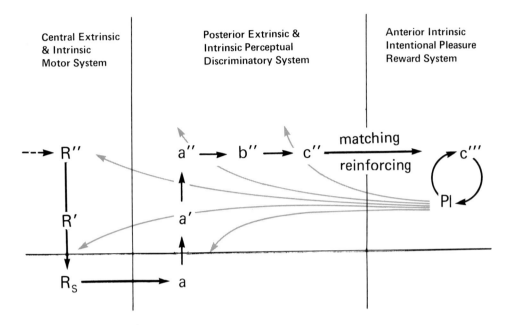

Figure XII-3. Reward reinforcement of a sensory-motor response as a function of expectation matching an activated Reward System representation.

The resultant increase in Pleasure-Reward System activation is shown as reinforcing the maintenance of the on-going response.

Postulates I and II may then be expressed in terms of reward effects upon sensory-motor behavior.

Postulate I

The maintenance and repetition of an initiated sensory-motor response R_s will be reinforced when that response results in a perception or perceptual expectation which matches an activated Pleasure-Reward System representation.

Postulate II

The maintenance and repetition of an initiated sensory-motor response will be disrupted or inhibited when that response interrupts a perception or perceptual expectation which was matching an activated **Pleasure-Reward System** representation.

Chapter XIII

The Anterior Intentional System
in Relation to
Voluntary and Goal-Directed Behavior

Anterior Intrinsic Upper Limbic Cortex:
The Concept of Wishes

According to the present neurophysiological model, upper limbic Pleasure System (c''' / Pl) processes are characterized by the following properties:

1. They are intimately involved with the arousal of pleasure and reward.

2. Once activated, they may be maintained by reverberatory processes for long periods of time.

3. They may be established by learning; the association of upper limbic representations with the Pleasure-Reward System may be conditional.

4. The matching of perception with a representation within the Pleasure System increases pleasure.

5. The interruption of perception matching a representation within the Pleasure System decreases pleasure.

The characteristics of these limbic system processes may be compared with those commonly associated with the concepts of "wishes," "intentions," "purposes," "goals," or "plans," which are generally recognized as having the following characteristics:

1. They are intimately involved with the arousal of pleasure and reward. Freud (1953:598) clinically arrived at this conclusion which became so basic to his theory: "A current of this kind in the apparatus . . . aiming at pleasure, we have termed a 'wish.'" To say, "What do you wish?" may be translated by "What would be your pleasure?"

2. They are generally considered as being able to be maintained for long periods of time.

3. They may be established by learning.

146

4. Perception matching a wish (wish-fulfillment or realization) is universally recognized as increasing pleasure.

5. The interruption of perception matching a wish is universally recognized as reducing pleasure (and heightening displeasure).

The characteristics common both to activated Pleasure System representations and to wishes are repeated for emphasis in Table XXVI.

This comparison leads to the proposal that a wish is the psychological counterpart of a physiological process involving a representation activated within the limbic Pleasure (Reward) System, 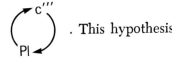 . This hypothesis

provides a basis whereby postulates I and II may be expressed in terms of wishes.

Differentiation of Terms

Although terms such as "wishes," "goals," "intentions," or "plans" are often used interchangeably, they focus upon different aspects of reaction. The term "wish" is used to refer more to emotional feelings, while the terms "intention" and "purpose" refer in particular to performance.

Cofer and Appley (1964:5) note in addition that the concept of "goal" puts the emphasis upon objects or situations in the environment, although it also includes some reference to the corresponding internal CNS mental representations of these objects or situations. In the field of behavioral

TABLE XXVI
A NEUROPHYSIOLOGICAL BASIS FOR WISHES

Upper Limbic Pleasure-Reward System Circuit Representational Processes	Wishes
1. Are intimately involved with eliciting pleasure and reward	1. Are intimately involved with eliciting pleasure and reward
2. May be maintained for long periods of time	2. May be maintained for long periods of time
3. May become established by learning	3. May become established be learning
4. Matched by perception increases pleasure	4. Matched by perception (wish fulfillment) increases pleasure
5. Interruption of matching with perception reduces pleasure (and heightens displeasure)	5. Interruption of matching with perception (interruption of wish fulfillment) reduces pleasure (and heightens displeasure)

*As formulated in relation to the present neurophysiological model.

psychology, interest has always been directed toward the concrete operational definition of terms and toward the observation of environmental events which may be controlled qualitatively and quantitatively. Therefore, behaviorists have preferred to deal with (1) a goal stimulus defined as a stimulus which has become associated with reward stimulus conditions (see Kimble, 1961:479, 484) rather than with (2) a CNS representation of a goal stimulus associated with a CNS reward system mechanism.

Despite these differences in emphasis, the concepts of an activated Pleasure-Reward System representation and a goal mechanism, wish, plan, or intention will be considered essentially equivalent. Postulate I then may be reduced to a behavioral concept that a goal, wish, plan, or intention matched by perception or expectation contributes to reinforcement of on-going behavior (Pribram, 1963:220–6).

These neurophysiological formulations pertaining to the interaction of perceptual and intentional systems as a basis for the cognitive selection of behavior were foreshadowed by E.C. Tolman (1932:10, 71, 76, 84, 95, 101, 162). Although Tolman's presentations were not always sharply defined, his experimental studies with animals and his theoretical conclusions regarding purposive behavior directed attention to the variables with which the present model has been concerned: Tolman concluded that the cognitive selection of behavior is a function of perception and perceptual expectation as they relate to the organism's goals.

Anokhin (1969:830–54) has carried out physiopsychological studies which have focused upon the role of goal variables interacting with discriminatory perception as a source for cognitive selection of voluntary behavior. Beritashvili (1969:660–1) concludes that goal-oriented behavior is controlled by images of the environment or by more complex plans. Cole and Maltzman (1969:33–5) note that this focus upon plans is directly in accord with Tolman's emphasis upon goals as a key to the understanding of voluntary behavior.

Chapter XIV

Cognitive Selection of Behavior:
Evidence from the Fields of
Clinical Neuropathology
and Cybernetics

Cognitive Selection of Behavior
A Function of Perception Matching Intentions;
Evidence from the Field of Clinical Neuropathology

The conclusion that cognitive selection of behavior is a function of matching posterior cortical perceptions with anterior cortical goals or intentions is substantiated by findings from the field of clinical neuropathology.

A.R. Luria (1964, 1966), at the University of Moscow, has studied the effects of cortical brain lesions involving the prefrontal[*] upper limbic cortex. He has employed psychological tests to evaluate the effects of such brain lesions upon behavioral performance. His findings indicate that the prefrontal processes are associated with the cognitive selection of performance as related to the matching of goals with the perception of behavior. Prefrontal (upper limbic) lesions therefore should interfere with this cognitive basis for the selection of behavior. Luria (1966:156) refers to these conclusions as follows: "Another important mechanism of the performance of purposive actions . . . is significantly impaired: A patient with a massive lesion of the frontal lobes very soon ceases to compare his performance of an action with his original plan, and he can no longer determine whether the action in fact, corresponds to the plan. Hence, such a patient, as a rule, does not rectify his mistakes and does not notice that his actions no longer conform to the original plan. As a result, the actions of a patient with a frontal lobe lesion, although intact with regard to their motor composition, easily lose their selective, purposive character and are converted into uncontrollable stereotypes." Luria (1964:355–6) points out "how easily the behavior of a patient with

[*] Luria uses the term "frontal" as an equivalent of "prefrontal."

149

a lesion of the frontal lobes loses goal-oriented character and becomes a series of isolated, immediate reactions to particular stimuli. . . ." And again (ibid:355), "Disturbances occurring after lesions of the frontal lobes often manifest themselves . . . as a loss of the controlling function of intentions or programs upon the behavior . . . a general loss of some feedback mechanism, a disturbance in signals of error, or an inadequate evaluation of the patient's own action. It can be reduced to a deficit in matching" (the perception of) "action . . . with the original intention. . . ."

Cognitive Selection of Behavior
A Function of Perception Matching Intentions; Evidence from the Field of Cybernetics

Cybernetics, the mathematical science of computers, is concerned not only with the functions of mechanical self-regulating machines but also with the functions of an animate self-regulating machine: the human nervous system. An understanding of the relevance of cybernetics to human brain functions requires a preliminary summary of some basic concepts pertaining to this field.

Webster's dictionary defines cybernetics as the comparative study of control systems. The term comes from the Greek word for governor or steersman. In other words, the field pertains to the study of selector systems which control, govern, or steer performance via the operation of selector or goal settings.

A cybernetic self-regulating machine contains mechanisms which provide for the following functions (Ashby, 1954:52–5): (1) the performance of responses which result in environmental change, (2) the registration of "feedback" of environmental change occurring during the machine's performance (ibid:37–9), (3) a concomitant registration of a "selector" or "goal" setting, (4) the matching of environmental feedback registration and selector-goal setting, (5) performance influenced by the equivalence or discrepancy between environmental feedback registration and selector-goal setting.

Ashby points out that a thermostatic heating control system offers the simplest example of self-regulating machine functions operating in accordance with cybernetic principles:

1. The *response-performance* of the thermostatic heating control system is mediated by the operation of the furnace motors providing for the release of heat.

2. The *registration of environmental temperature feedback* by the thermostatic control system is mediated by the operation of a simple thermometer.

3. Concomitant registration of a *"selector"* or *"goal"* *setting* within the thermostatic control system is mediated by mechanisms connected with the temperature dial-setting of the thermostat.

4. The *matching of environmental feedback registration and selector-goal-setting* within the thermostatic heating control system is mediated by the interaction of (a) actual temperature registration with (b) the dial-setting registration. The thermostat is affected by the difference between the registration of the actual and set temperatures.

5. The matched *equivalence* or *discrepancy* of the registration of environmental temperature with the selector-goal-setting exerts an influence upon on-going performance of the thermostatic heating control system: the thermostatic OFF switch is triggered when the position of the mercurial column registering temperature is equivalent to the selector-goal-setting. Conversely, the ON switch is triggered when the position of the mercurial column registering temperature is discrepant with (less than) the position of the temperature selector-goal-setting.

The operation of a thermostatic control system is represented in Figure XIV–1.

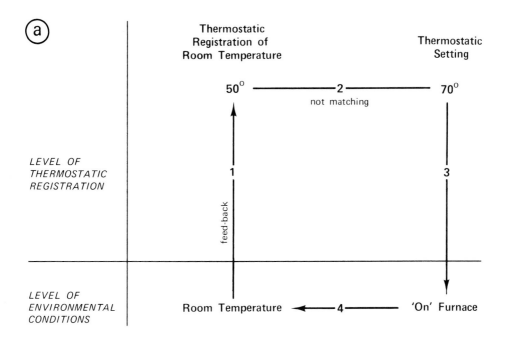

EAG

Figure XIV-1a. Operation of a thermostatic control system: registration of room temperature does not match the thermostatic setting.

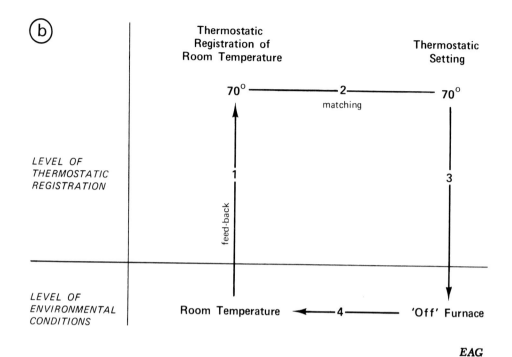

EAG

Figure XIV-1b. Operation of a thermostatic control system: registration of room temperature and thermostatic setting are matching.

The registration of the room temperature continues to be pitted against the thermostatic "goal" setting. As long as a discrepancy exists in which environmental temperature registration is less than the reading of the selector-goal-setting, the furnace motor will be activated. But, as soon as registration of room temperature matches, is equal to the selector-goal·setting, a different mechanism is released, and the furnace is turned off. Thus, the operation of a furnace thermostat describes a very simple example of equivalence-discrepancy selection of performance.

Attention becomes drawn to the parallel between (1) the functioning of the thermostat heating-control system according to the basic principles of cybernetics, and (2) the functioning of the neurophysiological model as developed within the preceding pages and presented in Figure XII–3. This model contains the basic mechanisms which are essential for the operation of a cybernetic self-regulating machine:

1. The *response-performance* of the neurophysiological model at hand is mediated by the initiation of response, via specific conditional $S \rightarrow R$ innervation or via non-specific activation of extrapyramidal rhythmic movements.

2. The *registration of environmental feedback* is mediated by the innervation of sensory discriminatory perception, ($\rightarrow c''$).

3. The concomitant registration of a *selector or goal setting* is mediated by innervation of reverberating Pleasure-Reward System circuit

representational processes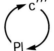

4. The *matching* of *environmental feedback registration* and *selector-goal-setting* is mediated by the interaction of the innervated perceptual processes with the activated reverberating Pleasure-Reward System rep-

resentational processes 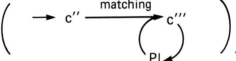 .

5. Matched *equivalence* of the environmental feedback registration and selector-goal-setting exerts an influence upon on-going performance: increased pleasure-reward activation during matched equivalence of perception and Pleasure-Reward System processes eventuates in maintenance of on-going performance.

Discrepancy of the environmental feedback registration with selector-goal-setting exerts an influence upon on-going performance: reduced pleasure-reward activation during discrepancy of perception and Reward System processes eventuates in disruption of on-going performance via the antithetical activation of the Punishment System. Behavior continues to be disrupted and changed until finally *matching* of perception and intention replaces mismatching, "discrepancy" or error. Consequent Reward System reactivation eventuates in the maintenance of the new behavior.

The comparisons presented in Table XXVII demonstrate that the mechanisms of this neurophysiological model essentially parallel those of the thermostatic heating-control system in meeting the cybernetic requirements for the operation of self-regulating machines:

TABLE XXVII*
THE PROPOSED NEUROPHYSIOLOGICAL MODEL AS COMPARED WITH A THERMOSTATIC HEATING-CONTROL SYSTEM

A
Pertaining to the Thermostatic-Heat-Control System

Registration of environmental temperature (feedback)	Not matching	Selector-goal temperature setting	Furnace motor ON
Registration of environmental temperature (feedback)	Matching	Selector-goal temperature setting	Furnace motor OFF

B
Pertaining to the Present Neurophysiological Model

Perceptual registration of environmental feedback	Matching	Goal representational setting	Reward System ON (non-specifically reinforcing concomitant response)
Perceptual registration of environmental feedback	Not matching	Goal representational setting	Reward System OFF (non-specifically disrupting concomitant response)

*The analogy becomes more exact when presented in terms of the Punishment System. See Appendix VI.

These conclusions coincide with Ashby's description of a self-regulating machine (see Cofer and Appley, 1964:346): "Reacting to . . . stimulation, the system . . . responds. Its response affects the environment in some particular way, at the same time 'reporting back' what has been done. The central regulatory apparatus then computes the discrepancy between performed and intended action, and the succeeding response is 'corrected for error.' "

In summary, the model's structure is based upon principles pertaining to the matching of perceptual and intentional processes and, in particular, to the matching of processes of the posterior perceptual and the anterior intentional systems of the cerebral cortex. These principles are in accord not only with the findings of neuroanatomy, neurophysiology, neuropathology, and experimental psychology, but also with the mathematical and experimental knowledge which has been derived from the cybernetic science of computer functions.

Bibliography

Adey, W.R., *et al.:* Effects of L-S-D-25 psilocybin and psilocin on temporal lobe EEG patterns and learned behavior in the cat. *Neurology, 12,* 1962.

Aichhorn, A.: *Wayward Youth,* rev. 2nd ed. New York: Viking, 1935.

Akert, K.: Comparative anatomy of frontal cortex and thalamofrontal connections. In Warren, J., and Akert, K.: *The Frontal Granular Cortex and Behavior.* New York: McGraw-Hill, 1964.

Altmann, Margaret: Naturalistic studies of maternal care in moose and elk. In Rheingold, H. (Ed.): *Maternal Behavior in Mammals.* New York: John Wiley, 1963.

Anokhin, P.K.: Cybernetics and the integrative activity of the brain. In Cole, M., and Maltzman, D. (Eds.): *A Handbook of Contemporary Soviet Psychology.* New York: Basic Books, 1969.

Arduini, A.: The tonic discharge of the retina and its central effects. In Moruzzi, G., Fessard, A., and Jasper, H. (Eds.): *Progress in Brain Research,* Vol. I, Brain Mechanisms. Amsterdam: Elsevier, 1963.

Arnold, M.: *Emotion and Personality,* Vol. II. New York: Columbia University Press, 1960.

Ashby, W.R.: *Design for a Brain.* London: Chapman and Hall, 1954.

Azrin, N., *et al.:* Intermittent reinforcement by removal of a conditioned aversive stimulus. *Science, 136,* 1962.

Beach, F.: Sexual behavior of prepuberal male and female rats treated with gonadal hormones. *J Comp Psychol, 34,* 1942.

Beach, F.: Instinctive behavior: reproductive activities. In Stevens, S.S. (Ed.): *Handbook of Experimental Psychology.* New York: John Wiley, 1951.

Beach, F.: Neural and chemical regulation of behavior. In Harlow, H.F., and Woolsey, C.N. (Eds.): *Biological and Biochemical Bases of Behavior.* Madison: University of Wisconsin Press, 1958.

Bechterew, W.: *Die Funktionen der Nervencentra.* Vol. 3. Jena: Gustav Fischer, 1911.

Bennett, A.M.H.: Sensory deprivation in aviation. In Solomon, P., *et al.* (Eds.): *Sensory Deprivation.* Cambridge, Mass.: Harvard University Press, 1961.

Beritashvili, I.S.: Concerning psychoneural activity of animals. In Cole, M., and Maltzman, I.: *A Handbook of Contemporary Soviet Psychology.* New York: Basic Books, 1969.

Bishop, M., Elder, S.T., and Heath, R.: Attempted control of operant behavior in man with intracranial self-stimulation. In Heath, R. (Ed.): *The Role of Pleasure in Behavior.* New York: Hoeber Medical Division, Harper and Row, 1964.

Boling, J.L., *et al.*: Post-parturitional heat responses of newborn and adult guinea pigs. Data on Parturition, *Proc Soc Exp Biol Med, 42,* 1939.

Bowers, C.Y., *et al.*: Porcine thyrotropin releasing factor vs. (pyro)glu-his-pro(NH₂). *Endocrinology, 86,* 1970.

Bowsher, D.: Termination of the central pain pathway in man: the conscious appreciation of pain. *Brain, 80,* 1957.

Brady, J.: The paleocortex and behavioral motivation. In Harlow, H., and Woolsey, C. (Eds.): *Biological and Biochemical Bases of Behavior.* Madison: University of Wisconsin Press, 1958.

Breder, C.M., and Coates, C.W.: Sex recognition in the guppy lebistes reticulatus. In Peters (Ed.): *Zoologica, 19,* 1935.

Breuer, J., and Freud, S.: Studies on hysteria. In *The Complete Psychological Works of Sigmund Freud,* standard ed., Vol. II. London: Hogarth, 1955.

Brookhart, J.: The cerebellum. In Field, J., Magoun, H.W., and Hall, V. (Eds.): *Handbook of Physiology, Section on Neurophysiology,* Vol. II. Washington, D.C.: Am Physiological Soc, 1960.

Brutkowski, S.: Prefrontal cortex and drive inhibition. In Warren, J., and Akert, K. (Eds.): *The Frontal Granular Cortex and Behavior.* New York: McGraw-Hill, 1964.

Bunn, J.P., and Everett, J.W.: Ovulation in persistent-estrous rats after electrical stimulation of the brain. *Proc Soc Exp Biol Med, 96,* 1957.

Burgus, R., *et al.*: Characterization of ovine hypothalamic hypophysiotropic TSH-releasing factor. *Nature, 226,* 1970.

Cannon, W.B.: Again the James-Lange and the thalamic theories of emotion. *Psychol Rev, 38,* 1931.

Cannon, W.B.: *The Wisdom of the Body,* 2nd ed. New York: Norton, 1939.

Cofer, C.N., and Appley, M.H.: *Motivation: Theory and Research.* New York: John Wiley, 1964.

Cole, M., and Maltzman, I: *A Handbook of Contemporary Soviet Psychology.* New York: Basic Books, 1969.

Crighton, D., Schneider, H.P.G., and McCann, S.M.: Localization of L-H releasing factor in the hypothalamus and neurohypophysis as determined by *in vitro* method. *Endocrinology, 87,* 1970.

Crosby, E., Humphrey, T., and Lauer, E.: *Correlative Anatomy of the Nervous System.* New York: Macmillan, 1962.

Cross, B.A., and Harris, G.W.: The role of the neurohypophysis in the milk-ejection reflex. *J Endocrinol, 8,* 1952.

Davidson, J.: Control of gonadotropin secretion in the male. In Martini, L., and Ganong, W. (Eds.): *Neuroendocrinology,* Vol. I. New York: Academic Press, 1966.

Delgado, J.M.R.: Limbic system and free behavior. In Adey, W.R., and Tokizane, T. (Eds.): *Progress in Brain Research,* Vol. 27, Structure and Function of the Limbic System. Amsterdam: Elsevier, 1967.

Delgado, J.M.R.: *Physical Control of the Mind.* New York: Harper and Row, 1969.

Delgado, J.M.R., Roberts, W.W., and Miller, N.E.: Learning motivated by electrical stimulation of the brain. *Am J Physiol, 179,* 1954.

Dell, P.: Reticular homeostasis and critical reactivity. In Moruzzi, G., Fessard, A., and Jasper, H.: *Progress in Brain Research,* Vol. I, Brain Mechanisms. Amsterdam: Elsevier, 1963.

DeLong, M.: Central patterning of movement. *Neuroscience Research Program Bulletin, 9,* 1971.

Dempsey, E., and Morison, R.: The production of rhythmically recurrent cortical potentials after localized thalamic stimulation. *Am J Physiol, 135,* 1942.

DeVore, G.: Mother-infant relations in free-ranging baboons. In Rheingold, H. (Ed.): *Maternal Behavior in Mammals.* New York: John Wiley, 1963.

Diamond, S., *et al.: Inhibition and Choice.* New York: Harper and Row, 1963.

Durup, G., and Fessard, A.: L'eletroencephalogramme de l'homme. *Annee Psychol, 36,* 1935.

Eldred, E.: Posture and locomotion. In Field, J., Magoun, H.W., and Hall, V. (Eds.): *Handbook of Physiology, Section on Neurophysiology,* Vol. II. Washington, D.C.: Am Physiological Soc, 1960.

Eldred, E., and Fujimori, B.: Relations of the reticular formation to muscle spindle activation. In Jasper, H., Proctor, L., Knighton, R., Noshay, W., and Costello, R. (Eds.): *Reticular Formation of the Brain.* Boston: Little, Brown, 1958.

Eliasson, S.: Central control of digestive function. In Field, J., Magoun, H.W., and Hall, V. (Eds.): *Handbook of Physiology, Section on Neurophysiology,* Vol. II. Washington, D.C.: Am Physiological Soc, 1960.

Elwers, M., and Critchlow, V.: Precocious ovarian stimulation following interruption of stria terminalis. *Am J Physiol, 201,* 1961.

Forman, D., and Ward, J.: Responses to electric stimulation of caudate nucleus in cats in chronic experiments. *J Neurophysiol, 20,* 1957.

French, J.D.: The reticular formation. In Field, J., Magoun, H.W., and Hall, V. (Eds.): *Handbook of Physiology, Section on Neurophysiology,* Vol. II. Washington, D.C.: Am Physiological Soc, 1960.

Freud, S.: *An Outline of Psychoanalysis.* New York: Norton, 1949.

Freud, S.: Project for a Scientific Psychology. In *Origins of Psychoanalysis.* London: Imago, 1954.

Freud, S.: The Interpretation of Dreams. In *The Complete Psychological Works of Sigmund Freud,* standard ed., Vol. V. London: Hogarth Press, 1953.

Freud, S.: Beyond the Pleasure Principle. In *The Complete Psychological Works of Sigmund Freud,* standard ed., Vol. XVIII. London: Hogarth Press, 1955.

Freud, S., and Breuer, J.: See Breuer, J., and Freud, S. 1955.

Gellhorn, E.: *Autonomic Imbalance and the Hypothalamus.* Minneapolis: University of Minnesota Press, 1957.

Gesell, A., and Amatruda, C.: *Developmental Diagnosis,* 2nd ed. New York: Hoeber Medical Division, Harper and Row, 1947.

Gloor, P.: Amygdala. In Field, J., Magoun, H. W., and Hall, V. (Eds.): *Handbook of Physiology, Section on Neurophysiology*, Vol. II. Washington, D.C.: Am Physiological Soc, 1960.

Grastyan, E.: The hippocampus and higher nervous activity. In Brazier, M. (Ed.): *The Central Nervous System and Behavior*. Josiah Macy Jr. Foundation. Madison, N.J.: Madison Printing Co., 1959.

Green, J.: The hippocampus. In Field, J., Magoun, H.W., and Hall, V. (Eds.): *Handbook of Physiology, Section on Neurophysiology*, Vol. II. Washington, D.C.: Am Physiological Soc, 1960.

Greenacre, P.: Fetishism. In Freud, A., et al (Ed.): *Psychoanalytic Study of the Child*, Vol. VIII. New York: International Universities Press, 1953.

Greenacre, P.: Problems of infantile neurosis: a discussion. In Freud, A. (Ed.): *Psychoanalytic Study of the Child*, Vol. IX. New York: International Universities Press, 1954.

Grossman, S.P.: *A Textbook of Physiological Psychology*. New York: John Wiley, 1967.

Harlow, H.F.: The nature of love. *Am Psychol, 13*, 1958.

Harlow, H.F., and Harlow, M.K.: Social deprivation in monkeys. *Sci Am, 207*, 1962.

Harlow, H., Harlow, M., and Hansen, E.: The maternal affectional system of rhesus monkeys. In Rheingold, H. (Ed.): *Maternal Behavior in Mammals*. New York: John Wiley, 1963.

Harris, G.W.: Central control of pituitary secretion. In Field, J., Magoun, H.W., and Hall, V. (Eds.): *Handbook of Physiology, Section on Neurophysiology*, Vol. II. Washington, D.C.: Am Physiological Soc, 1960.

Hartmann, H., Kris, E., and Lowenstein, R.: Notes on the theory of aggression. In *Psychoanalytic Study of the Child*, Vol. III-IV. New York: International Universities Press, 1949.

Head, H.: *Studies in Neurology*, Vol. II. London: Oxford University Press, 1920.

Heath, R.: *Studies in Schizophrenia*. Cambridge, Mass.: Harvard University Press, 1954.

Heath, R.: Pleasure response of human subjects to direct stimulation of the brain: physiologic and psychodynamic considerations. In Heath, R. (Ed.): *The Role of Pleasure in Behavior*. New York: Hoeber Medical Division, Harper and Row, 1964.

Heath, R., and Gallant, D.: Activity of the human brain during emotional thought. In Heath, R. (Ed.): *The Role of Pleasure in Behavior*. New York: Hoeber Medical Division, Harper and Row, 1964.

Hebb, D.O.: *Organization of Behavior*. New York: John Wiley, 1949.

Hebb, D.O.: Alice in wonderland or psychology among the biological sciences. In Harlow, H.F., and Woolsey, C.N. (Eds.): *Biological and Biochemical Bases of Behavior*. Madison: University of Wisconsin Press, 1958.

Hefferline, R., et al.: Escape and avoidance conditioning in human subjects without their observation of the response. *Science, 130*, 1959.

Hernández-Péon, R., and Chavez-Ibarra, G.: Sleep induced by electrical or chemical stimulation of the forebrain. *Electroencephalogr Clin Neurophysiol Suppl, 24,* 1963.

Hernández-Péon, R.: Attention, sleep, motivation, and behavior. In Heath, R. (Ed.): *Role of Pleasure in Behavior.* New York: Hoeber Medical Division, Harper and Row, 1964.

Heron, W.: Cognitive and physiological effects of perceptual isolation. In Solomon, P., *et al.* (Ed.): *Sensory Deprivation.* Cambridge, Mass.: Harvard University Press, 1961.

Hersher, L., Richmond, J., and Moore, A.U.: Maternal behavior in sheep and goats. In Rheingold, H.L. (Ed.): *Maternal Behavior in Mammals.* New York: John Wiley, 1963.

Hess, W.R.: *Diencephalon, Autonomic and Extrapyramidal Functions.* New York: Grune and Stratton, 1954.

Hess, W.R.: *Bertrage zur Physiologie d. Hernstammes I. Die Methodik der lokalisierten Reizung und Ausschaltung subkortikaler Hernabschnitte.* Leipzig: Georg Thième, 1932.

House, E.L., and Pansky, B.: *A Functional Approach to Neuroanatomy,* 2nd ed. New York: McGraw-Hill, 1967.

Hydén, H.: The question of a molecular basis for the memory trace. In Pribram, K., and Broadbent, D. (Eds.): *Biology of Memory.* New York: Academic Press, 1970.

Ingram, W.R.: Central autonomic mechanisms. In Field, J., Magoun, H.W., and Hall, V. (Eds.): *Handbook of Physiology, Section on Neurophysiology,* Vol. II. Washington, D.C.: Am Physiological Soc, 1960.

Jasper, H.: Reticular-cortical systems and theories of the integrative action of the brain. In Harlow, H., and Woolsey, C. (Eds.): *Biological and Biochemical Bases of Behavior.* Madison: University of Wisconsin Press, 1958.

Jasper, H.: Unspecific thalamocortical relations. In Field, J., Magoun, H.W., and Hall, V. (Eds.): *Handbook of Physiology, Section on Neurophysiology.* Vol. II. Washington, D.C.: Am Physiological Soc, 1960.

Jasper, H., and Rasmussen, T.: Studies of clinical and electrical responses to deep temporal stimulation in man with some considerations of functional anatomy. In Solomon, H., Cobb, S., and Penfield, W. (Eds.): *The Brain and Human Behavior.* Research Publication of the Assoc for Research in Nerv and Mental Disease, Vol. XXXVI. Baltimore: Williams and Wilkins, 1958.

John, E.R.: *Mechanisms of Memory.* New York: Academic Press, 1967.

Jung, R., and Hassler, R.: The extrapyramidal motor system. In Field, J., Magoun, H.W., and Hall, V. (Eds.): *Handbook of Physiology, Section on Neurophysiology,* Vol. II. Washington, D.C.: Am Physiological Soc, 1960.

Kaada, B.: Cingulate, posterior orbital anterior insular and temporal pole cortex. In Field, J., Magoun, H.W., and Hall, V. (Eds.): *Handbook of Physiology, Section on Neurophysiology,* Vol. II. Washington, D.C.: Am Physiological Soc, 1960.

Kappers, A., Huber, G.C., and Crosby, E.: *The Comparative Anatomy of the Nervous System of Vertebrates Including Man,* Vols. I, II, III. New York: Hafner, 1936.

Kawakami, M., *et al.*: Mechanisms in the limbic system controlling reproductive functions of the ovary. In Adey, W.R., and Tokizane, T. (Eds.): *Progress in Brain Research,* Vol. 27, Structure and Function of the Limbic System. Amsterdam: Elsevier, 1967.

Kimble, G.: *Hilgard and Marquis' Conditioning and Learning,* 2nd ed. New York: Appleton-Century-Crofts, 1961.

Kluver, H., and Bucy, P.: Preliminary analyses of functions of the temporal lobes in monkeys. *Arch Neurol Psychiat, 42,* 1939.

Kluver, H.: Functional significance of the geniculo-striate system. In Kluver, H. (Ed.): *Visual mechanisms,* Lancaster, Pa.: J. Cattell, 1942.

Konorski, J.: *Integrative Activity of the Brain.* Chicago: University of Chicago Press, 1967.

Krieg, W.: *Functional Neuroanatomy.* Bloomington, Ill.: Pantagraph, 1966.

Kruger, L.: The thalamic projection of pain. In Knighton, R., and Dumke, P. (Eds.): *Pain.* London: Churchill, 1966.

Langworthy, O.R., and Richter, C.P.: Increased spontaneous activity produced by frontal lobe lesions in cats. *Am J Physiol, 126,* 1939.

Lashley, K.S.: *Brain Mechanisms and Intelligence.* Chicago: University of Chicago Press, 1929.

Lilly, J.: Learning motivated by subcortical stimulation: the start and stop patterns of behavior. In Jasper, H., *et al.* (Eds.): *Reticular Formation of the Brain.* Boston: Little, Brown, 1958.

Lilly, J.: The psychophysiological bases for two kinds of instincts. *J Am Psychoanal Assoc, 8,* 1960.

Lindsley, D.: Emotion. In Stevens, S.S. (Ed.): *Handbook of Experimental Psychology.* New York: John Wiley, 1951.

Lindsley, D.: Attention, consciousness, sleep and wakefulness. In Field, J., Magoun, H.W., and Hall, V. (Eds.): *Handbook of Physiology, Section on Neurophysiology,* Vol. III. Washington, D.C.: Am Physiological Soc, 1960.

Lindsley, O.R.: Operant behavior during sleep: a measure of the depth of sleep. *Science, 126,* 1957.

Lorente de Nó, R.: In Fulton, J.F. (Ed.): *Physiology of the Nervous System.* New York: Oxford Press, 1938.

Lorenz, K.: Companionship in bird life. In Schiller, C. (Ed.): *Instinctive Behavior.* New York: International Universities Press, 1957.

Luria, A.R.: *Human Brain and Psychological Processes.* New York: Harper and Row, 1966.

Luria, A.R., and Homskaya, E.D.: Disturbance in the regulative role of speech with frontal lobe lesions. In Warren, J.M., and Akert, K. (Eds.): *The Frontal Granular Cortex and Behavior.* New York: McGraw-Hill, 1964.

MacLean, P.: New findings relevant to the evolution of psychosexual functions of the brain. *J Nerv Ment Dis, 135,* 1962.

MacLean, P.: Phylogenesis. In Knapp, P. (Ed.): *The Expression of the Emotions in Man.* New York: International Universities Press, 1963.

MacLean, P., and Delgado, J.M.R.: Electrical and chemical stimulation of frontotemporal portion of the limbic system in the waking animal. *Electroencephalogr Clin Neurophysiol*, 5, 1953.

MacLean, P., and Ploog, D.: Cerebral representation of penile erection. *J Neurophysiol* 25, 1962.

MacLean, P., Denniston, R., and Dua, S.: Further studies on cerebral representation of penile erection: causal thalamus, midbrain and pons. *J Neurophysiol*, 26, 1963.

MacLean, P., and Creswell, G.: Anatomical connections of visual system with limbic cortex of monkey. *Comp Neurol*, 138, 1970.

Magoun, H.W.: Non-specific brain mechanisms. In Harlow, H., and Woolsey, C. (Eds.): *Biological and Biochemical Bases of Behavior*. Madison: University of Wisconsin Press, 1958.

Mangili, G., Motta, M., and Martini, L.: Control of adrenocorticotropic hormone secretion. In Martini, L., and Ganong, W. (Eds.): *Neuroendocrinology*, Vol. I. New York: Academic Press, 1966.

Meites, J.: Control of mammary growth and lactation. In Martini, L., and Ganong, W. (Eds.): *Neuroendocrinology*, Vol. I. New York: Academic Press, 1966.

Meites, J., and Sgouris, J.: Effects of altering the balance between prolactin and ovarian hormones on initiation of lactation in rabbits. *Endocrinology*, 55, 1954.

Mittelmann, B.: Motility in infants, children and adults: patterning and psychodynamics. In *Psychoanalytic Study of the Child*, Vol. IX. New York: International Universities Press, 1954.

Morison, R.S., and Dempsey, E.W.: A study of thalamo-cortical relations. *Am J Physiol*, 135, 1942.

Moruzzi, G., and Magoun, H.: Brain-stem reticular formation and activation of the EEG. *Electroencephalogr Clin Neurophysiol*, 1, 1949.

Moruzzi, G.: Spontaneous and evoked electrical activity in the brain-stem reticular formation. *XX Int Physiol Congr, Abstr of Rev*, 1956.

Nauta, W.: Hypothalamic regulation of sleep in rats, an experimental study. *J Neurophysiol*, 9, 1946.

Nauta, W., and Kuypers, H.: Some ascending pathways in the brain stem reticular formation. In Jasper, H., Proctor, L., Knighton, R., Noshay, W., and Costello, R. (Eds.): *Reticular Formation of the Brain*. Boston: Little, Brown, 1958.

Nauta, W.: Some efferent connections of the prefrontal cortex in the monkey. In Warren, J., and Akert, K. (Eds.): *The Frontal Granular Cortex and Behavior*. New York: McGraw-Hill, 1964.

Noordenbos, W.: Some aspects of anatomy and physiology of pain. In Knighton, R., and Dumke, P. (Eds.): *Pain*. London: Churchill, 1966.

Oberholzer, R.J.H, and Tofani, W.O.: The neural control of respiration. In Field, J., Magoun, H.W., and Hall, V. (Eds.): *Handbook of Physiology, Section on Neurophysiol*, Vol. II. Washington, D.C.: Am Physiological Soc, 1960.

Olds, J.: Adaptive functions of paleocortical and related states. In Harlow, H., and Woolsey, C. (Eds.): *Biological and Biochemical Bases of Behavior*. Madison: University of Wisconsin Press, 1958.

Olds, J.: The mechanisms of voluntary behavior. In Heath, R.G. (Ed.): *The Role of Pleasure in Behavior*. New York: Hoeber Medical Division, Harper and Row, 1964.

Olds, J., and Milner, P.: Positive reinforcement produced by electrical stimulation of septal area and other regions of rat brain. *J Comp Physiol Psychol, 47*, 1954.

Oswald, I.: *Sleeping and Waking*. Amsterdam: Elsevier, 1962.

Pampiglione, G., and Falconer, M.: Electrical stimulation of the hippocampus in man. In Field, J., Magoun, H., and Hall, V. (Eds.): *Handbook of Physiology, Section on Neurophysiology*, Vol. II. Washington, D.C.: Amer Physiological Soc, 1960.

Papez, J.W.: A proposed mechanism of emotion. *AMA Arch Neurol Psychiat, 38*, 1937.

Penfield, W., and Boldrey, E.: Somatic motor and sensory representation in the cerebral cortex of man as studied by electrical stimulation. *Brain, 60*, 1937.

Penfield, W., and Perot, P.: The brain's record of auditory and visual experience, a final summary. *Brain, 86*, 1963.

Pfaffman, C.: The sense of taste. In Field, J., Magoun, H.W., and Hall, V. (Eds.): *Handbook of Physiology, Section on Neurophysiology*, Vol. I, Washington, D.C.: Am Physiological Soc, 1959.

Pribram, K.: Neocortical function in behavior. In Harlow, H., and Woolsey, C. (Eds.): *Biological and Biochemical Bases of Behavior*. Madison: University of Wisconsin Press, 1958.

Pribram, K.: The intrinsic systems of the forebrain. In Field, J., Magoun, H.W., and Hall, V. (Eds.): *Handbook of Physiology, Section on Neurophysiology*. Vol. II. Washington, D.C.: Am Physiological Soc, 1960.

Pribram, K.: The neuropsychology of Sigmund Freud. In Bachrach, A.J. (Ed.): *Experimental Foundations of Clinical Psychology*. New York: Basic Books, 1962.

Pribram, K.: A neuropsychological model: some observations on the structure of psychological processes. In Knapp, P. (Ed.): *Expression of the Emotions in Man*. New York: International Universities Press, 1963.

Rasmussen, A.T.: Effects of hypophysectomy and hypophysial stalk resection on the hypothalamus nuclei of animals and man. *Res Publ Assoc Res Nerv Ment Dis, 20*, 1940.

Reese, E.: *The Analysis of Human Operant Behavior*. Dubuque, Iowa: William C. Brown, 1966.

Ribble, M.: *The Rights of Infants*, 2nd ed. New York: Columbia University Press, 1965.

Rose, J.E., and Woolsey, C.N.: Organization of the mammalian thalamus and its relationships to the cerebral cortex. *Electroencephalogr Clin Neurophysiol, 1*, 1949.

Rose, J., and Mountcastle, V.: Touch and kinesthesis. In Field, J., Magoun, H.W., and Hall, V. (Eds.): *Handbook of Physiology, Section on Neurophysiology*, Vol. I. Washington, D.C.: Am Physiological Soc, 1959.

Ruch, T., Patton, H., Woodbury, J.W., and Towe, A.: *Neurophysiology*, 2nd ed. Philadelphia: Saunders, 1965.

Sawyer, C.: Reproductive behavior. In Field, J., Magoun, H.W., and Hall, V. (Eds.): *Handbook of Physiology, Section on Neurophysiology*, Vol. II. Washington, D.C.: Am Physiological Soc, 1960.

Scheibel, M., and Scheibel, A.: Structural substrates for integrative patterns in the brain stem reticular core. In Jasper, H., *et al.* (Eds.): *Reticular Formation of the Brain*. Boston: Little, Brown, 1958.

Shadé, J.P.: The limbic system and the pituitary-adrenal axis. In DeWied, D. (Ed.): *Progress in Brain Research*, Vol. 32, Pituitary, Adrenal, and the Brain. Amsterdam: Elsevier, 1970.

Sperry, R.W.: Physiological plasticity and brain circuit theory. In Harlow, H., and Woolsey, C. (Eds.): *Biological and Biochemical Bases of Behavior*. Madison: University of Wisconsin Press, 1958.

Stamm, J.: The function of the median cerebral cortex in maternal behavior of rats. *J Comp Physiol Psychol, 48*, 1955.

Strom, G.: Central nervous regulation of body temperature. In Field, J., Magoun, H.W., and Hall, V. (Eds.): *Handbook of Physiology, Section on Neurophysiology*, Vol. II. Washington, D.C.: Am Physiological Soc, 1960.

Sweet, W.: Pain. In Field, J., Magoun, H.W., and Hall, V. (Eds.): *Handbook of Physiology, Section on Neurophysiology*, Vol. I. Washington, D.C.: Am Physiological Soc, 1959.

Szentagothai, J., *et al.: Hypothalamic Control of the Anterior Pituitary*. Budapest: Akademiai Kiado, 1962.

Talbot, S., and Marshall, W.H.: Physiological studies on neural mechanisms of visual localization and discrimination. *Am J Ophthalmol, 24*, 1941.

Tolman, E.C.: *Purposive Behavior in Animals and Men*. New York: Appleton-Century-Crofts, 1932.

Tseng, F.: Differentiation of anger and fear in the emotional behavior of the rat. Unpublished MA thesis, University of Toronto, 1942.

Urquhart, J.: Neuroendocrine transducer input-output relations. *Neurosciences Research Program Bulletin, 9*, 1971.

Van Hoesen, G., Pandya, D., and Butters, N.: Cortical afferents to the entorhinal cortex of the rhesus monkey. *Science, 175*, 1972.

Walker, A., and Weaver, T.: Ocular movements from the occipital lobe in the monkey. *J Neurophysiol, 3*, 1940.

Walker, A.E.: Internal structure and afferent-efferent relations of the thalamus. In Purpura, D., and Yahr, M. (Eds.): *The Thalamus*. New York: Columbia University Press, 1966.

Watanabe, S., and McCann, S.M.: Localization of FSH-releasing factors in the hypothalamus and neurohypophysis as determined by *in vitro* assay. *Endocrinology, 82*, 1968.

Woodworth, R.S.: *Experimental Psychology*. New York: Holt, 1938.

Woolsey, C.N., and Walzl, E.M.: Topical projection of nerve fibers from local regions of the cochlea to the cerebral cortex of the cat. *Bull Johns Hopkins Hospital, 71,* 1942.

Woolsey, C., Marshall, W.H. and Bard, P.: Representation of cutaneous tactile sensibility in the cerebral cortex of the monkey as indicated by evoked potentials. *Bull Johns Hopkins Hospital, 70,* 1942.

Yakovlev, P., Locke, S., and Angevine, J.: The limbus of the cerebral hemisphere, limbic nuclei of the thalamus, and the cingulum bundle. In Purpura, D., and Yahr, M. (Eds.): *The Thalamus.* New York: Columbia University Press, 1966.

Young, P.T.: *Motivation and Emotion, a Survey of the Determinants of Human and Animal Activity.* New York: John Wiley, 1961.

Appendix I

Freud's Concepts as Related to Non-specific Activation Theory

As early as 1893 Breuer and Freud's (1955:198) description of "intra-cerebral tonic excitation" foreshadowed current descriptions of ascending tonic non-specific arousal activation of consciousness and wakefulness. Breuer wrote: "We may also assume that there is an optimum for the height of the intracerebral tonic excitation. At that level of tonic excitation, the brain is accessible to all external stimuli, the reflexes are facilitated, though only to the extent of normal reflex activity, and the store of ideas is capable of being aroused and open to association in the mutual relation between individual ideas which corresponds to a clear and reasonable state of mind. It is in this state that the organism is best prepared for work." Breuer and Freud also wrote of localized attention as a function of a non-uniformity in the distribution of intracerebral tonic excitation (ibid:195).

In a similar vein, Freud (1954:397–9) anticipated non-specific activation theory as he wrote of diffuse cathexis* of perception as a determinant of consciousness, sleep and attention. He referred to sleep (ibid: 398) as a lowering of the endogenous cathexis charge of the psyche, while "hypercathexis" (1953:594) was responsible for attention. Freud's emphasis on cathexis, Pribram (1962:445) writes, "is one of those strokes of luck or genius which in retrospect appears uncanny for only in the past decade have neurophysiologists recognized the importance of the graded non-impulsive activities of neural tissue, graded mechanisms such as those of dendritic networks whose functions are considerably different from those of transmitted impulse activity of axons."

* James Strachey, who edited Freud's *Outline of Psychoanalysis,* (1949:23, fn) wrote: "The words 'cathexis' and 'to cathect' . . . are terms with which Freud expresses the idea of psychical energy being lodged in or attaching itself to mental structures or processes, somewhat on the analogy of an electric charge."

Expectation in Relation to Spatial
as Well as Temporal Distribution of Stimuli

The processes of expectation involve a part, or one component of a stimulus sequence, specifically reactivating the representation of the total sequence. If the presentation of one component, a, of a *temporal* series a — b — c may elicit the representation of the total sequence a″→b″→c″, then the presentation of one component of a *spatial* stimulus series a — b — c should also be able to elicit the representations of the total sequence a″ → b″ → c″. If a vase, a lamp, and a clock are seen always together on a certain table, one speaks of "expecting" to see the lamp when one sees only the vase and the clock.

The processes whereby perceptual spatial expectations are elicited by the presentation of one or more components of a total stimulus configuration, provide a basis for understanding the Gestalt phenomenon of "closure". This may prove essentially to be a manifestation of the establishment of spatial or temporal expectation whereby the presentation of a part, a, of the total spatial or temporal configuration will tend to elicit

not only the perception 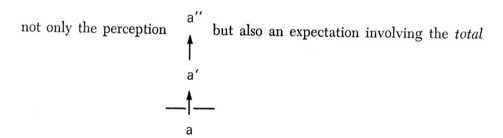 but also an expectation involving the *total*

spatial configuration,

Conjoint Functions of Extrinsic and Intrinsic Sensory Cortices: Verbal Perception and Associations

The auditory perception of a spoken word may be schematically represented as follows:

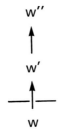

where w, w′ and w″ symbolize respectively a spoken word and its extrinsic and intrinsic sensory representations. More exactly,

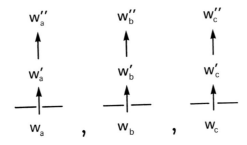

denote the perceptions of words w_a, w_b, and w_c.

In such a case

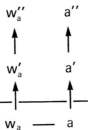

denotes the process of pairing perception of word, w_a, with perception of object, a, a basis for the association of intrinsic (gnostic) representations w_a'' and a'':

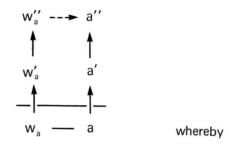

whereby

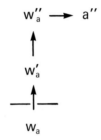

or expressed linearly:

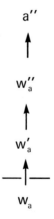

In a similar fashion, word w_b may become associated with and elicit the intrinsic representation, b'', of object b:

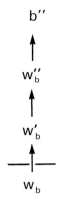

Therefore the pairing of the words w_a — w_b eventuates in

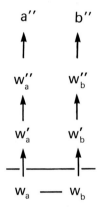

serving the association not only of intrinsic word representations w_a'' and w_b'' but also of a'' and b'':

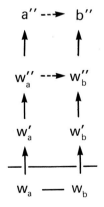

According to this formulation, the association of intrinsic representations $a'' \rightarrow b''$ may be attained either directly via paired presentation of actual events, $a - b$:

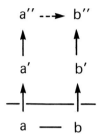

or indirectly via the paired presentation of the words w_a (which had been associated with, a), and of w_b (which had been associated with, b):

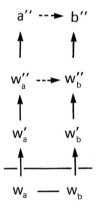

In this way, words (w_a, w_b, etc.,) and their perceptions are in a position to contribute to the association of intrinsic thoughts:

$$\boxed{a'' \;\rightarrow\; b''}$$

and since

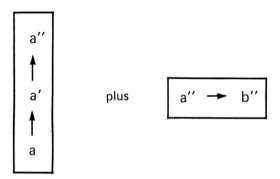

results in the formation of expectation

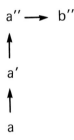

this expectation may be derived from the presentation of the words w_a and w_b even though actually, a, may never have been followed by, b.

Additional Cognitive Sources of
Pleasure and Unpleasure

The symbolic reasoning by which hypotheses have been derived with respect to perception or expectation matching Pleasure System circuit

representations,  may be applied toward the derivation of a cor-

responding set of hypotheses that pertain to perception or expectation

matching Unpleasure System circuit representations

1. If perception matches an activated Unpleasure System circuit representation (a "dislike"):

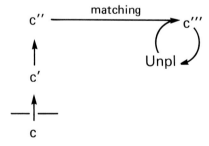

then, theoretically, the Unpleasure System should be charged:

$$c \longrightarrow c' \longrightarrow c'' \xrightarrow{\text{matching}} c''' \longrightarrow \text{Unpl}$$

2. Likewise, if expectation matches an activated Unpleasure System circuit representation:

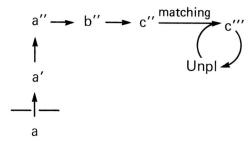

then once again, the Unpleasure System should be charged:

$$a \longrightarrow a' \longrightarrow a'' \longrightarrow b'' \longrightarrow c'' \longrightarrow c''' \longrightarrow Unpl$$

3. Conversely, interruption of perception or of expectation matching an activated Unpleasure System circuit representation should charge the reciprocally antithetical Pleasure System:

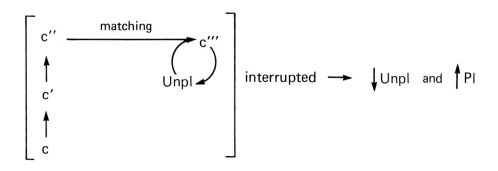

Cognitive Sources for Charging
The Pleasure (Reward) System
A Schematic Model

The following schematic diagrams illustrate in slow motion picture fashion how the innervation of a perception or perceptual expectation *matching* an activated Pleasure System circuit representation may charge the non-specific Pleasure System.

Within the diagrams, red lines refer to circumstances during which certain cortical connections, established in the past, are being specifically innervated. Gray lines refer to circumstances during which the same connections are not being innervated.

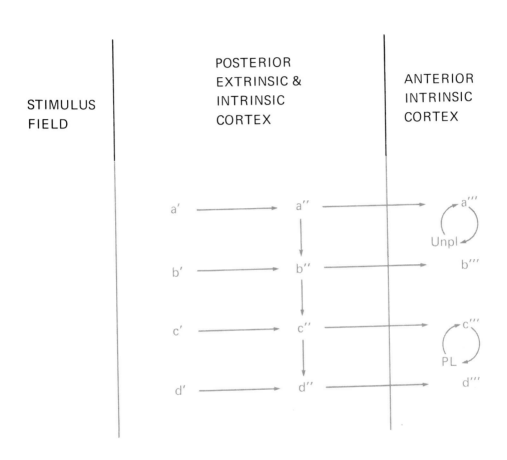

Figure AV-1. Connections have already become established but at the moment are not being specifically innervated.

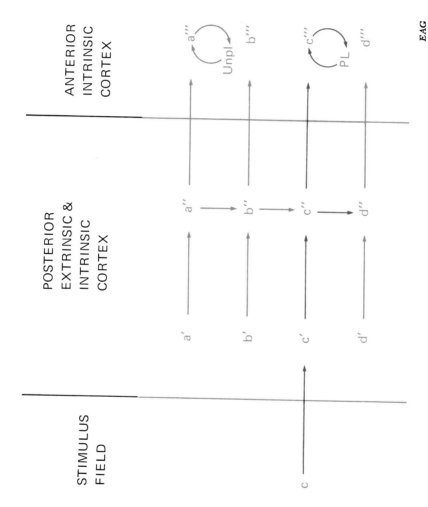

Figure AV-2. Presentation of stimulus c innervates the already established connections c → c′ → c″ thereby specifically activating perception of c. These processes charge the Pleasure System circuit

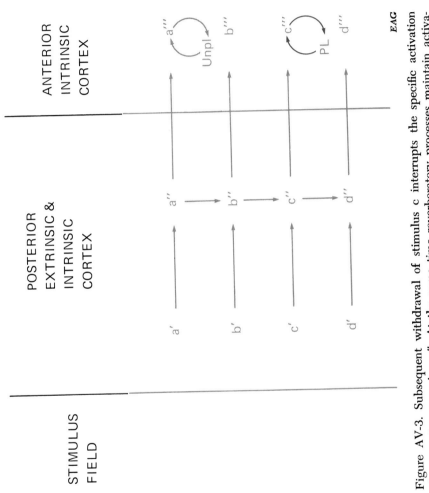

Figure AV-3. Subsequent withdrawal of stimulus c interrupts the specific activation of perception c → c′ → c″. At the same time reverberatory processes maintain activa-

tion of the Pleasure System circuit

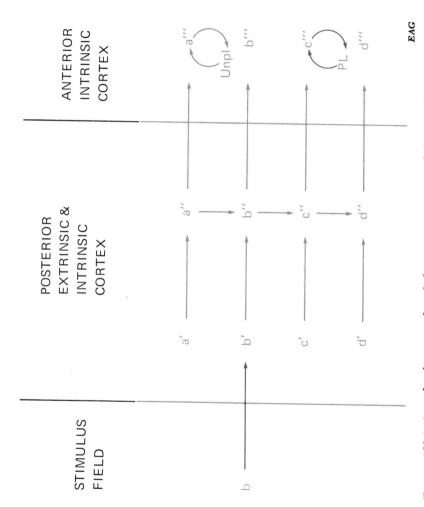

Figure AV-4. Stimulus b is introduced during continuation of the reverberatory processes activating

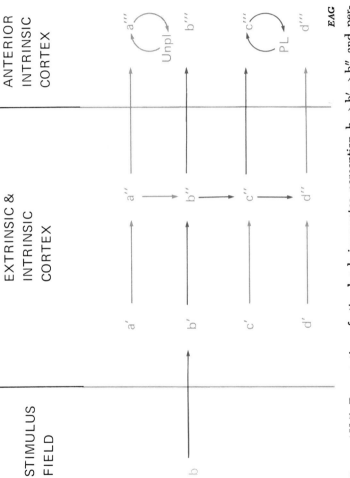

Figure AV-5. Presentation of stimulus b innervates perception $b \rightarrow b' \rightarrow b''$ and perceptual expectation $b \rightarrow b' \rightarrow b'' \rightarrow c''$. Reverberatory processes continue to maintain

the activation of the Pleasure System circuit ⟳ . At such a time the *innervated*

perceptual expectation, $\rightarrow c''$ *matches the specifically activated Pleasure System Circuit*

representation, ⟳ *thereby facilitating* Pleasure System charge via the specifi-

cally activated series $b \rightarrow b' \rightarrow b'' \rightarrow c'' \rightarrow c''' \rightarrow Pl$.

TABLE XXVIII
THE PROPOSED NEUROPHYSIOLOGICAL MODEL AS COMPARED WITH
A THERMOSTATIC HEATING-CONTROL SYSTEM

A
Pertaining to the Thermostatic-Heat-Control System

Registration of environmental temperature (feedback)	Matching	Selector-goal temperature setting	Furnace motor OFF
Registration of environmental temperature (feedback)	Not matching (less than)	Selector-goal temperature setting	Furnace motor ON

B
Pertaining to the Present Neurophysiological Model

Perceptual registration of environmental feedback	Matching	Goal representational setting	Punishment System OFF*
Perceptual registration of environmental feedback	Not matching	Goal representational setting	Punishment System ON†

*Reward System ON

†Reward System OFF

Author Index

181

Subject Index